RAISING
RYLAND

RAISING RYLAND

OUR STORY OF PARENTING A TRANSGENDER CHILD WITH NO STRINGS ATTACHED

HILLARY WHITTINGTON

WITH KRISTINE GASBARRE

wm

WILLIAM MORROW

An Imprint of HarperCollinsPublishers

HarperCollins books may be purchased for educational, business, or sales promotional use. For information please e-mail the Special Markets Department at SPsales@harpercollins.com.

FIRST EDITION

Designed by Diahann Sturge

Library of Congress Cataloging-in-Publication Data has been applied for.

ISBN 978-0-06-238888-9

16 17 18 19 20 OV/RRD 10 9 8 7 6 5 4 3 2 1

For Ryland and Brynley, with hopes of making this world a more loving, accepting place for you and the future generations to thrive

Contents

Author's Note

This is a work of nonfiction. The events and experiences detailed herein are all true and have been faithfully rendered as we have remembered them, to the best of our ability. Some names, identities, and circumstances have been changed in order to protect anonymity of the various individuals involved. Though conversations come from our keen recollection of them, they are not written to represent word-for-word documentation; rather, we've retold them in a way that evokes the real feeling and meaning of what was said, in keeping with the true essence of the mood and spirit of the event.

Please note that in the first chapter, when this story starts, we will refer to Ryland using female pronouns. Then, at the point in the story when we allow Ryland to transition to the male gender, we will use male pronouns, which everyone who knows him does today.

Prologue

"Mom . . . why did God make me this way?"

It happened two years ago, but I still remember it like it was yesterday: in his Batman zip-up pajamas and with his chin quivering, five-year-old Ryland stood in the doorway of his bedroom. His face streamed with tears as he looked up at me, struggling to understand why he'd been the kid chosen to walk such a difficult road.

It's amazing how one question can hold the power to change everything in your life. It was profound in its simplicity, and the most incredible part of it was the fact that it came from a toddler. But that's who Ryland is: the innocent, self-aware, strong, and compassionate child who has already educated millions of people about what it means to be transgender.

The moment when I knew we could not ignore Ryland's journey had actually occurred the night before he asked me that question, after he'd told me that he would wait for our family to die so he could cut his hair. To him, only being free of the very people who loved him most would make it possible for him to exist on the outside as the same person he was on the inside.

It's hard for most people to imagine that starting as young as age two, a child could feel so much anguish about being categorized as one gender when he identified with the other. As parents, it's our job to guide our children into making healthy, wise decisions for their future; but few parents ever face the degree of challenges that we've experienced with Ryland. As devastated as we were to get the diagnosis that our child was deaf, just after his first birthday, no one could have prepared me for the news that this same child, my little Ryland, was also transgender.

But there was no fighting it. At two years old, Ryland underwent a procedure to receive cochlear implants that made it possible for him to hear. But almost as soon as he was able to hear our words and communicate with us verbally, he needed us to listen to the truth that he was trying to express: "I'm a boy," our child would tell us, even though Ryland had been assigned female at birth.

It grew impossible to try to talk him out of it. After much conflict, many sleepless nights, and stacks of books written by developmental psychologists, gender experts, and individuals who had made their own gender transitions, we knew that we had to allow our daughter to become our son.

This was our child, and we would love Ryland unconditionally, but our fears came from how the *world* would view our child. Wearing external devices on each ear that make it possible for the cochlear implants to do their job, Ryland was already *visibly* different . . . but as the reality of our child's gender identity grew clear, I didn't want Ryland to go through the pain of *feeling* different. As his mother, when I read the statistic that 41 percent of transgender people attempt to take their own lives by age twenty, I felt speechless—but it ignited a certain empowerment in me. Prior to that, I'd been lost, but now I had direction. I would *not* lose *my* child this way . . . even if that meant sacrificing my marriage to the man I loved—Ryland's father, Jeff.

Through it all, however, we remain together, and Ryland's knowledge of who he is never wavers. This is part of what many people find so lovable and admirable about him.

Raising Ryland is our story of raising a child who lives with not one, but *two* factors that have threatened to make him an outcast in today's world. Primarily, this book chronicles our journey as a family with a child who has voluntarily stepped up before the public in an effort to bring understanding to the plight of the seven hundred thousand Americans, plus those unknown numbers of people, who are transgender like him. Our goal in writing this book is to let them know that they are not alone—that there is love here for them.

We're also eager to bring more understanding about this topic to all families, teachers, and individuals who are open and even interested to learn more about it. We're not here to single-handedly sway all of society to accept Ryland and the transgender population. Instead, we're here as a mother and a father who are determined to do everything we can to create an environment where our child can grow up with the chance to cultivate the same self-love and confidence to which every child has the right when he or she is born.

This book is also the revelation of the private turmoil we have faced as the parents of a transgender child, the resistance we've encountered from some of our family, the overwhelming amount of love and support that pours in to us from friends and strangers, and our commitment to our mission to make the world a better, more loving place for both of our children—Ryland and his little sister, Brynley.

Denial is the most common way for parents of transgender children to deal with the signs we noticed early on . . . and most transgender children are not as fortunate as Ryland is. Having known what the book is about when you picked it up, readers might marvel at the irony that we encountered as we recalled some of the early events of Ryland's life—before we were aware that on the inside, our child was a boy. Most transgender children don't have parents who accept them and embrace them for who they really are. For us, and for those children, it's time to uncover the truth. There are many transgender children in this world who will become part of that terrifying statistic.

Ryland is one of the lucky few who can be himself. We wouldn't have it any other way.

Part One

Learning to Listen

Chapter One

Ryland's Creation

I'm not looking for love on the Fourth of July in 2003, but, as they say, that's exactly when you find it.

In June 2003, I ended a year-long relationship with a boy I met during my sophomore year at the University of California, San Diego. Like me, he was a communications major, but unlike me—who has found an internship at a local news station here at home—he's taken off for the summer in New York to pursue his dreams of finding work in theater.

My friend Tammy, an upbeat coworker at a local chain restaurant, has made a summer project of helping to get me over my heartbreak. I have to give her credit—she's doing a great job. "Oh good," she says as I climb into her passenger's seat.

"What's good?"

"You're in flip-flops. We'll have to park and walk awhile."

Pacific Beach is one of the most happening spots in all of San Diego, especially on the height of summertime holidays. After we find parking, it takes us thirty minutes on foot to make our way to the sand. We're sweltering by the time we spot the roped-off property that a group of friends from work has reserved. When a round of margaritas makes it our way, Tammy and I toast and giggle over the first salty sip.

I scan the scene: thousands of young, excitable, beautiful people packed up and down the San Diego coast. Around us, they laugh and dance and pose for photos.

Then, my eyes land on a group standing next to us—good-looking guys, all tan and fit. My eyes fix on one in particular: he's tall with dark hair, green eyes, and muscular, broad shoulders. He's gorgeous.

I lean into Tammy. "Look at him," I say.

"The one in the gray T-shirt? *Yeah*. I know."

"No," I point, inconspicuously. "The taller one."

Just then, he glances over.

"He just caught me pointing!" I whisper. Tammy and I burst out laughing. Secretly, I'm glad he busted me.

Gradually, his group hovers in to circle around ours, and he and I begin to chat. His name is Jeff, he tells me. He's twenty-six, five years older than I am, and has just finished his master's degree in industrial technology at Cal Poly, on the central coast. He's been working as an EMT and doing some real estate on the side with his dad, but he's considering going into a field where he can be hands-on in helping people full-time—paramedic training, the fire academy, or maybe even medical school.

Instantly, I'm intrigued.

I like Jeff's ambition and the fact that he likes to be the one helping people—our attraction is instant and mutual. The ocean water is warm and glimmering with sunshine when he invites me to join him for a swim, but after a few minutes, his friends holler down to him—they're leaving to host a house party that night. I follow his lead out of the water and whisper to Tammy, who's waiting at my towel: "We have to join them." Fortunately, she and Jeff's friend have hit it off, too.

When we arrive, his smile lights something inside me: *This is what they mean when they talk about love at first sight.* As he and I stay close at the party and talk, it's clear that he's ready for the same things I've always dreamed of: to find someone to share life with, to share a home and start a family.

The first few dates solidify my feelings for Jeff. I open up to tell him about the problems in my family, mainly my older brother, who's been struggling with a serious drug problem since we were teenagers. Jeff listens quietly, with great patience and understanding, and when he responds, he's thoughtful, kind, and intelligent. He's the eldest of three boys, very responsible, and he loves to take charge and manage everything. Jeff always chooses the right thing to do, and over time, I find a deep sense of security in him. He's the first man who's ever made me feel safe—an experience I have never felt in my life, definitely not in dating. I trust him to make sure nothing bad will happen to me—to protect me.

Over the next couple of months, I grow more and more sure that Jeff is everything I've ever wanted in a man, but because I know right away that I'm going to marry him, I can feel myself coming on too strong—and so can he. He's used to being a bachelor who lives on the beach, and I observe that maybe he would prefer to remain free to do whatever he wants.

Three months into our relationship, in October, Jeff's birthday arrives. Not knowing where we stand or whether he wants me to be part of it, I decide to break things off. I tell him that if someone doesn't reciprocate my feelings, I can only continue to give for so long. Because I can't be completely cruel, I leave the gift that I'd bought him—a surf shirt—outside his door.

Hurt and angry, he calls me. "Why did you do this?" I know he's referring to both the gift and the breakup. Gently, I tell him that I really care about him, but that I need things to be different if he wants me in his life.

He goes out and buys himself a new truck—a man's rebellious manner of coping with heartbreak—and within a couple of weeks, he picks me up in his truck and asks for reconciliation. He says he regrets letting me get away and makes a decision to open up more and commit. I'm not sure that he's ready to change so for the next few weeks I tread very lightly and maintain some distance from him . . . but, unable to imagine my future with anyone else, I finally decide to give him another chance.

Right away, I begin to see Jeff including me into more of his life. A month later, on Thanksgiving, he takes me to meet his parents. On the wall inside their hallway, he points out a portrait of his family. There are dozens of them, and they're all handsome and pulled together. By the way Jeff talks about them, I sense that he will make an amazing father someday.

But following that day, there's one piece that's still holding him back: he speaks often about the need for a bigger challenge in his life; more incentive to work harder and use the gifts God gave him. He's decided that he wants to join the fire department and train as a paramedic, and I support him to move forward with the decision—even taking on some of the costs of his tuition.

The week of my college graduation in June 2004, just shy of a year since we met, Jeff proposes. I'm beside myself. We nail down some of the details immediately: the date, which will be July 2005, the ceremony's location on the beach, and Pastor Eric—the former pastor of the church where I grew up, which is an hour north of where we live in San Diego—to perform our wedding. Pastor Eric is a longtime friend of our family, and he commits to our wedding date and leads us through our preparations when we drive up to see him for premarital counseling. The session between the two of us and Pastor Eric confirms that I have made the right choice in my future husband—we share the same beliefs about love, family, and faith, and Jeff has Pastor Eric's seal of approval as well as my dad's. It doesn't get any more assuring than that. Besides having a home and a family, I can't imagine what our future might hold, but if it includes Jeff, I'm ready for anything.

As I browse wedding blogs and magazines, I can only wish for the stresses that most other brides seem to face: *How to pare down the guest list? Which colors to put on the bridesmaids?*

My biggest worry in our wedding planning isn't a factor I've ever been able to control—it's my brother. The opinion of Jeff's family means a lot to me, and there's been a struggle in my life that's been the source of deep shame for years. My brother, Ryan, is two years older than I am. He lives in Oregon on some property our grandfather owned, but even when he's away, I worry about him constantly. He has such a great capacity for love that his sensitivity is sometimes too much for him to bear, and for the better part of the last decade, Ryan has suffered a serious substance abuse problem.

He's my only sibling, and he and I are very close. Recently I even bought him a journal. *I wish I could be up there when you need me,* I wrote on the front page, *but if you ever can't get a hold of me and need to talk, just jot down your thoughts in this little book.*

Of course I want my brother *at* my wedding, but I just don't know whether it's a good idea to put him *in* the wedding. For Ryan to be a central part of the celebration, inside a mix of strangers and alcohol on a very emotional day, could be a recipe for embarrassment in front of my new in-laws.

To help me decide, I turn to Jeff. He knows how much my brother means to me deep down, and tells me, "We have to include him, Hill. You'll always regret it if you don't."

Jeff's wisdom and compassion in such a touchy situation cause me to fall even deeper in love with him, and soon, on July 9, 2005, our wedding day arrives. Showing up in his linen grooms-man suit, combed hair, and clean-trimmed goatee, Ryan cooperates beautifully, posing in all of our bridal party photos with a proud smile and participating cheerfully in the festivities. Later, my parents tell me that as they were driving my brother to the airport, he told them: "Hillary's wedding was the best day of my life."

At the time, none of us knows that it will also be one of the last days of his life.

THE FIRST YEAR following our wedding isn't exactly the way I'd imagined. With most of our finances going toward Jeff's training at the fire academy for the city of San Diego, I return to the restaurant where I worked with Tammy and pick up as many shifts as I can. I crave something more: I've always been drawn to high-stress environments—it's why I wanted to be a television news reporter. Now, as a new wife in her early twenties, I'm beginning to wonder whether I'll ever be able to pursue the dreams I had for my own life.

I begin to consider going back to school for nursing, but our lifestyle ends up taking priority. After our wedding, we rented a two-story beach house in Pacific Beach, just three blocks from the sand. The house is one of the most amazing designs I've ever seen, complete with secret passages and artsy designs crafted into every corner. We frequently entertain friends and spend our money going out to eat, and it's not long before our finances have spun us into a panic. Jeff and I sit down and have a very honest discussion: I'd always believed that getting married was supposed to create security, and deep down, I'm feeling resentment at Jeff. How is it fair for him to pursue his passions, while I pay a majority of the bills? We agree that we have to start prioritizing better, and we need to make some sacrifices—together. We look long term. What are our dreams? We want to have children, we want to buy a home, and to do either or both of these, we need to start saving money.

When our one-year lease is up, we pack up the little furniture we have and put it into storage. Then we move out of our beach house, and in with Jeff's parents, fifteen miles east of the beach in the suburbs of Mount Helix. As a temporary plan, I cannot complain—it's generous of them to let us move in on their space, and my mother-in-law keeps a home and a yard that could be featured in *Better Homes & Gardens*. I can hardly enjoy it, though. I'm so worried about what my in-laws think of me, and I feel devastated—humiliated—that at twenty-four years old, I cannot take care of myself financially. In our bedroom, Jeff and I often argue in a forced hush, and I feel like a failure to both him and his parents. There's no one I can vent to in private, and I never thought that even with a husband, it would still be possible to feel alone in the world.

After a few weeks, we're having so much trouble that we decide to take some time apart. I pack a bag and leave for the weekend to stay with a waitress friend, who takes me to a party and reminds me how to let loose like I haven't done since college. We arrive back at her apartment in a blur and fall asleep for a little while . . . until late that night—August 12, 2006—when my life changes forever.

It's my cell phone that wakes me up, my dad's number on the glowing display. It's also two o'clock in the morning. "Hillary?"

"Dad?"

"There's been an accident."

I grip the V-neck of my pajama top as my dad's voice shakes while he narrates the details: my brother had been at a party, and, after drinking too much, he got behind the wheel of a car. Then he and two of his friends—one of them who was in my class, she's the young mother of an infant—tried to make it home. "Someone is dead, Hill, but they won't tell us who. Mom and I are headed to the scene now."

"No . . ."

"Hillary . . ."

"I'm coming home!"

I hang up and run into the bathroom, where I lose everything I've consumed throughout the course of the night. Then I emerge, and I call Jeff's phone. . . .

No answer.

I dial again, but still, there's no answer, and again. I leave a message. "My brother's been in an accident, Jeff, someone's dead. Please call me back!"

After a couple of minutes, my phone rings. He's with friends around a bonfire on the beach, and he's had some drinks, too. "I don't know what's happening, Jeff."

"I'm coming up there. Let me call your folks," he says, and when he does, he can hear the emotion in my father's voice.

"They won't let us on the scene, Jeff, they won't tell us anything!"

"Tim," Jeff tells my dad, "if he's alive, he needs you at the hospital—not there. Hillary is on her way to your house. I'll sit tight here until she arrives there, so I can talk you through this. Just do me a favor and keep me posted."

My friend and I call a taxi and head an hour north, straight to my parents' house in Lake Elsinore.

When my parents get to the hospital, they call Jeff again.

"Jeff," Dad says. "We're at the hospital."

"And?"

"Jeff . . . he's not here." There's some commotion, so they get off the line and a few minutes later, my dad calls Jeff again. My dad's friend is a retired California highway patrolman and he has gained access to the scene. "Jeff," my dad says through tears. "It's him."

THE SUN IS rising when we leave to visit the accident scene. In the middle of the night, Jeff's parents drive him up to my parents' house and pick up my best friend, Renee, on the way. En route to the scene, Jeff turns to me while we're sitting at a stoplight. "Babe," he says. "I've been thinking. We should honor your brother by naming our firstborn after him."

I look into his eyes, knowing what this means—we're staying together—and wanting him to know that he's just given me something more meaningful than I've ever experienced before. From this point, a child might be the one thing that can pull me out of what lies ahead.

When we reach the scene, the morning sun is in full blaze. A group has formed—among us, Renee and my cousin Melissa, whom I grew up with and who, from now on, will be the closest thing I have to a sibling. If there's anyone here who can relate to the depth of my grief, it's her.

The emergency responders have left. Jeff is busy staking a cross in the ground. Melissa, who's a nursing student, is well accustomed to offering comfort in painful moments. She and Renee stay close behind me as I search the vicinity of the crash site for the last pieces of my brother's life. Tossed in a bush, I locate one of his green flip-flops . . . and as I scan my eyes some more, I see the last evidence of his life: a puddle of blood, still wet, on a pile of gravel specked with broken glass. I've fallen to my knees when Jeff comes to my side. "What is that?" he says.

I show him my finger, now painted red. "It's his blood," I tell him. "It's still wet." Sobs overtake me, and I collapse onto the ground. I lift my face and through my tears, I seek out any glimpse of comfort—then there, in the distance, beyond the highway, the image strikes me: the old stone building with its clay-tile roof—the church where my family and I used to attend church on Sundays.

The feeling rushes back to me, how as small children my brother and I would turn around in our pew to watch my parents play the bells in the choir loft. At the front of the church was always Pastor Eric, playing his guitar for all of us children during the Sunday services. Even as I sit here now, I can hear Pastor Eric sing the words of my favorite song:

This is the day that the Lord has made.
I will rejoice and be glad in it.
This is the day, this is the day that the Looooord has made . . .

But when Pastor Eric left the church, so did our family. It was right around the same time that my brother started getting into trouble and my dad was working hard to provide. As a family, we lost touch with spirituality.

I grasp for the peace and happiness I used to feel when Pastor Eric was on the altar; that calming time in my life when I was free from worry and heartache. I think of Ryan, how recently he had finally listened to me and returned to church when he moved back home from Oregon. He began to volunteer his time at the church and wore his name badge proudly. I was so proud, and relieved, when he told me that he'd been growing close with the clerical staff and was looking to the pastors for some positive influence in his life.

And here, in this moment at the place where my brother has died, it dawns on me that I haven't seen Pastor Eric since right after our wedding. There was always something about Pastor Eric that made me feel an innate sense of peace, regardless of what was going on. Even my brother agreed—in his final effort to try to clean up his life, Ryan had written in his journal that he intended to make more of an effort to talk to God and the pastors at church.

By now, Jeff has approached me. He peels me up from the side of the highway. "We have to go, honey," he says. "Traffic is slowing down for us. This isn't safe."

For the next few days, I eat nothing. I stay at my parents' home, with its revolving door of visitors and a blur of funeral arrangements and tasks to complete. My mom sits limp and helpless on the couch, while my dad entertains the countless visitors in a way that makes me wonder if he's even aware that my brother is gone.

Jeff stays with me, losing sleep right alongside me. Lying next to him, I realize: How dare I consider giving up on him? How dare I accuse him of letting me down? This is my husband. We made a pledge for forever. Life can change in an instant, and here I've been, worrying about something so insignificant as money and my pride. Thank God we have family we can turn to, I realize. Thank God his parents were willing to take us in and help care for us when we were just learning to take care of each other.

DAYS AFTER THE funeral, I return to stay with Jeff and his parents. I also call the restaurant and quit my job. In the weeks to follow, I find it difficult to get out of bed. Jeff leaves every morning for the fire academy and doesn't return until late in the evenings. On the rare occasion that I leave the bedroom we occupy, my mother- and father-in-law sometimes exchange worried glances. One day shortly after Ryan's funeral, Jeff's dad knocks and enters our bedroom, where I lie hidden under the covers in my pajamas.

"Come on, Hill," he says. I pull the covers down from over my head and meet his gaze in the morning light. "Get out of your pajamas. You're coming with me." His voice is stern and strong, not at all like his usual easygoing, upbeat tone.

"Where are we going?"

"We're going to run some errands together. You can't stay in bed like this."

In his car, we head for La Mesa, an area just a few minutes away from Mount Helix. "So . . ." I say casually. "What's going on?"

"Peg and I have been talking, Hill," he says.

"You have?" I hold my breath, thinking he's about to tell me that they're finished helping us; that I'm a useless partner to their son and that Jeff and I are on our own if we want to try to stay together.

"Yes, we have. We want to help you and Jeff get on your way."

I turn and look at him, his blue eyes shining in the light that's streaming through the car's windows.

"I want you to start working with me," he says. "Maybe that will help you start saving again. It's time you two start thinking about having a home—I'll help you find one, you know."

"Rand, you will?"

"Of course! After all, Peg and I want some grandkids!"

Right then, I realize that a smile has spread across my face, something I haven't felt in weeks.

We spend every evening for the next couple of weeks searching the Internet for a perfect property for Jeff and me. Then we find one, a condo with a comfy living area and just enough space for us to grow. When we go to view it, Jeff and I smile at each other: it's the perfect size for a young family.

We make our offer and Rand orchestrates the entire transaction—a lifesaver, since Jeff is gone all day at the fire academy.

Later that week, Rand gets the news: the owners have accepted our offer. A few weeks after we move in, we rescue a young white-and-tan boxer . . . and we start trying to have a baby.

Trying, I say, because it doesn't come easily. With Jeff's schedule at the fire department and the fact that I've taken a job from one of Rand's friends, a dentist, who offered me a full-time opportunity to help run his office, we both could do with a little more time and energy. Plus, with the weight of losing my brother, my emotional stress has confused my body out of its normal cycle. After about six months of unsuccessful attempts, we see a fertility specialist, who determines there's nothing wrong with either of us—it's just all about timing. Hearing me express how much I want this baby, a friend at work lends me her expensive ovulation monitor, and within a month, I can feel that something is very different.

It's April 23, 2007, when I learn that I'm pregnant. Kobe, our dog, is the first one to learn the news when I scream out loud and jump in the car to find Jeff at the fire station. "He's at a different house today!" his friend Jason yells from the fire station garage.

"Of course he is!" I laugh, and when I finally track him down near a station in the next district, he jumps off the engine to greet me.

"What's up, babe?"

"Here." I hand him an envelope with the pregnancy test strip and the answer key from the box inside. I let him figure out the results on his own. I watch his face as he interprets that two parallel pink lines indicate *Positive.*

He looks up at me, making sure he's read it right. "Hill," he says. "Are you serious?"

I nod.

He hugs me in the middle of the street and hollers to his guys. "We're having a baby!"

My doctor gives us a due date of the day after Christmas, and I start a journal, keeping track of all my symptoms and the emotions that are building inside me for our baby. I also browse baby information sites incessantly and sign up to receive weekly emails from one website that informs me week by week how our little one is growing. I'm amazed that at nine weeks, the baby's tiny limbs have formed, and at the start of the second trimester, his or her fingerprints have already developed—proof to the rest of the world what Jeff and I already know: that this child is one of a kind. A few weeks later, the baby's skeleton is transforming from delicate cartilage to more durable bone, and he or she can actually hear what's happening outside the womb. Apparently, the baby's hearing in utero is extremely sensitive, but by the time he or she is born, loud noises won't sound disturbing anymore.

By midsummer, around eighteen to twenty weeks along, we'll be able to learn the baby's gender. When anyone asks us which of the two we're hoping for, our answer is uniform and unison: it doesn't matter what we get. We just want a healthy baby.

The developments are exciting, but there are aspects of this baby's arrival that I struggle with. My emotions on most days are amplified by the fact that Jeff is rarely home to comfort me, and he wants me to keep working when the baby arrives, an idea that I cannot accept. I'm one of the only moms-to-be I know, and I acknowledge that I need to reach out to the few moms in our circle of friends. At a Memorial Day picnic, I confide in Michelle, the wife of one of Jeff's high school friends, telling her that I can't keep up with how I feel myself changing, physically or emotionally.

"Listen," she says. "When I was pregnant with Ethan, I felt like I couldn't relate to anyone. But can I tell you something?"

"What?"

"It's like this: you spend nine months dreaming about what this little person will be like, but then when he arrives, he's even more amazing than you've imagined."

"Really?"

"Oh, totally. You two were made to be parents, Hill. And I know it's tough right now when you're worried about money and trying to make big decisions . . . but you'll see, it all falls into place."

"I needed to hear that."

"I promise," she says. "Jeff will be an incredible father."

Michelle's advice helps me to enjoy the next few weeks, and at our next doctor's appointment, we have the chance to learn the baby's gender. "You want to know?" the doctor says.

Jeff and I look at each other. "Definitely."

ON JULY 30, 2007, we send out an email:

> It's a little girl!!!!
> Due: day after Christmas 2007
> Current length: 9 inches
> Weight: 0.5 lbs

We include the sonogram image of Ryland, and immediately, the responses begin to appear in my inbox. Michelle's is the first, saying, "I love it! Think of all the pink, the mom-daughter shopping days, a partner to lay out at the beach with . . . while I'll be here playing with worms and Transformers. Peg must be so excited too after three boys!"

Jeff's college buddy Zach—a father of two girls—writes from where he lives in Northern California. (He responds swiftly, as he and Jeff have been brainstorming a surf trip to Indonesia.) "Why is it the bad-asses like Jeff and me end up with girls? Just kidding. Little girls are spectacular.—Zach"

My mom's best friend, also a fire wife, writes to me after she hears the news: "Guess I'll have to start looking for pink fire engines!!!!!!"

During the weekends when Jeff is working around the clock, my mom makes the drive down to San Diego to keep me company, help with chores, and get my input for the November baby shower she's hosting for me back home. She also helps me decorate the nursery, which Jeff and I have painted in a soothing sage green with clean white trim and white furniture. We hang white letters on the wall that each hang from pink satin ribbons to spell: R-Y-L-A-N-D.

However, just as I'm settling into my third trimester in early October, Jeff is called out to deal with a storm of wildfires burning out of control in San Diego. We're instructed not to go outside because the air quality is so low, and I experience constant anxiety about my husband's safety—except for a twenty-four-hour break at home after five days, he works nonstop for more than a week. I'm starting to realize that with Jeff working in this field, I'll worry like this until he retires.

Again, our usual inner circle calls and writes to check in on us: my parents, Jeff's brothers and his friend Zach, and Michelle, whose family was evacuated from their home because the fires were spreading near their area. Peg and Rand check in on me often to make sure I'm hanging in there, but with everything I'm hearing on the news, my panic is growing.

Finally, the stress catches up with me when eight weeks before Ryland is scheduled to arrive, I go into preterm labor.

My doctor gives me two injections to stop the contractions and sends me home, where I'll be on bed rest for the next eight weeks, or as long as we can possibly keep the baby from coming.

Every few hours, I have to take a pill, which causes debilitating headaches and brings on jitters as if I've had twenty cups of coffee. The worst part is so bad that it's almost comical: I can't climb the stairs to our bathroom, so I keep a bucket next to me on the couch. My parents come down to stay with me, bringing me a wheelchair so that at least I can go outside for some fresh air. Together we all decide that it's best to cancel the baby shower that my mom planned. The good news is that for a few weeks, we're successful at controlling the contractions.

I study the baby development email updates religiously. The second week of November, one reads: "If you've been nervous about preterm labor, you'll be happy to know that babies born between 34 and 37 weeks who have no other health problems generally do fine. They may need a short stay in the neonatal nursery and may have a few short-term health issues, but in the long run, they usually do as well as full-term babies." This reassures me slightly, and my doctor echoes the same prediction: if we can make it to thirty-six weeks, he says, we will almost certainly be safe.

When Jeff is home, there's so much I'd love for us to be doing to prepare for the baby, but he insists that I stay put and let him take care of me. As I watch him around the house, there's a tiny little piece of me that would love to keep this man all to myself forever, but in our conversations with each other, we're both counting down the days until Ryland arrives and our life changes from a couple into a family.

Chapter Two

Baby Signs

My birthing video is recorded in the same spirit that I suspect every birthing video ever made has been shot: from behind the camera, my dad films a joyous anticipation in the delivery room the night before our first child, and the first grandchild on both sides, will arrive. I'm sure any parent can relate to the raw, humorous, occasionally intense moments throughout the video . . . but looking back, there was some remarkable foreshadowing about Ryland's life from even before birth.

The video begins early on the evening of Friday, November 30, 2007. In all of the preterm labor worries of these last couple of months, two of the things we felt very sure about were that we wanted to document the live birth, and we wanted to know the baby's gender beforehand. One of those decisions was easy, cut-and-dried.

The other will come to carry more significance in our lives than we know is possible at that time.

In the video, Jeff—wearing a plaid ball cap and a hooded sweatshirt—supervises the situation with the calmness, control, and optimism that caused me to fall in love with him. Behind him are chatter and laughs from my parents, Jeff's parents, and Jeff's brother Scott, who had moved home to San Diego from San Francisco in time for Ryland's arrival. Scott is loyal, level-headed, and revered as the family peacemaker among his two brothers. Scott is also gay, and thanks in part to the fact that my father-in-law's sister is a lesbian and a longtime LGBTQ activist, the family has embraced Scott with pure love. I do, too—he's one of my best friends. Occasionally, I have even accompanied him on nights out to the gay bars in Hillcrest, the neighborhood in San Diego that's known for its diversity, love, and acceptance.

There are moments captured in the video that have persisted throughout my experience as Ryland's mother. "There's Hillary, the proud mother!" my dad says at one point when I'm in labor, while at another point I say to my doctor: "I'm in a lot of pain. Is this normal?" A few minutes later, my dad announces his good-natured intention to turn off the camera to conserve the battery "until the real heavy stuff comes," he says—*the real heavy stuff* a reference to the pushing that was ahead very early the next morning. But none of us could have anticipated how heavy some parts of our future would be.

Next comes the magical moment. I had always imagined that my child would come out screaming, but in the video, for a few seconds after Ryland arrives, she actually remains peaceful, allowing the nurse to suction out her mouth a few times, before she finally releases a muscle of a cry. With tears, I laugh as they hand my baby to me. "Oh my God!" I kiss her. "*Ohmygodohmygod!*"

As the doctor stitches me up, our family all enters the room again while Jeff comforts me and scratches my scalp through my hair. "You're so strong," he says, kissing my head. "You did it."

And then in the background, there is a moment of question among two nurses, one of whom has just arrived to start the morning shift. "Is it a boy or a girl?" she asks.

"It is . . ." The nurse who had suctioned Ryland's mouth pauses as if to check the chart; as if twenty seconds ago, the bottom of a baby girl hadn't been turned up at the world as they bundled her up for me to hold her. "A girl."

Every time I watch the video, I remember how surreal it was for me to hear the voice of the little human whose whole entire life until minutes before had taken place silently, inside me. When I witness the experience now, more than seven years later, I remember the sheer awe I felt with every sound she made as soon as she entered the world. *How long has she had that voice?* I wondered. *What is she trying to tell us?*

Indeed, from the very beginning, there were some very important things that Ryland needed us to know.

The first instance of real concern comes just a few minutes later. "I think she's a little sleepy from having the umbilical cord around her neck," says another nurse. I look at my mom, then my dad, then at Jeff's family. There's an alarmed silence in the room, and when the nurse registers our responses, she jumps in with a further explanation to alleviate our worry. "It takes them a minute," she says. "She's alert and crying and everything, but we'd just like her to be a little more alert. We have high expectations." We all laugh, softened with the relief of her levity. "She just dropped onto the planet, and we want it all."

Ryland coughs, then cries. I look at the camera, then to Jeff. "Is she okay?" I ask him.

"I *think* so," he says.

And like so many parents before us, we both turn to her expectantly, trying to decipher the mystery of what her cries are telling us.

FOR THE FIRST year after Ryland's arrival, I sometimes joke that I feel as though my life is like *Groundhog Day*. Almost the moment that we arrive home from the hospital, Jeff agrees with me that it would be best for me to stay at home with the baby . . . but because of what that means for us financially, he works around the clock to make ends meet.

In the mornings, I feed Ryland and do things around our condo—Kobe always on my heels, seeking more attention than I have the hands to give him. When I'm cooking or just standing back to watch her, Ryland plays with toys in the living room—always drawn to those with motion or flashing lights, like the fire truck my parents bought for her. Its siren wails throughout the condo so loudly that I'm concerned we're bothering the neighbors, but Ryland absolutely loves the red light as it swirls around the plastic dome.

I feed her and walk her in the stroller to the supermarket to grab groceries for dinner, cooking giant meals to spoil Jeff when he gets home from working his second job, which he's secured to help make us a little extra money.

"How was your day?" he asks after he's taken a few minutes to unwind, and I tease him.

"Same as yesterday," I sigh, then break into a grin. He knows nesting like this is exactly what I wanted.

These nights, we often catch ourselves standing together over Ryland and staring in awe of her perfection—those dimpled cheeks she gets from her dad that turn to two shiny apples when she smiles, the way her eyes squint when she giggles wildly as Jeff blows raspberry kisses on her neck, her chubby little fists resting peacefully on her belly when she sleeps. I dress her the way I'd always dreamed of dressing a baby girl, in ruffles and flowers and shades of pink as soft as her little lips. We take pictures and videos almost daily and then entertain ourselves for hours by watching them over and over after we've put her down.

In the summer of 2008, Jeff's college buddies beg him to join them on their surf trip to Indonesia—"We need a paramedic with us, we've all pitched in for him to come!" Zach, the "badass" with two little girls, pleads to me.

"Honey," I tell him.

"I know, I know . . ." he says. "We have an eight-month-old, I can't leave you."

"No. What I was going to say is, I think you should go."

"Really?" His eyes are as wide as Ryland's are whenever I blow bubbles from the wand on the front porch . . . then his expression changes, as if he's hesitant. "You're sure?"

"I'm very sure," I tell him, wrapping my arms around his waist. "You work hard for us, and this is the trip of a lifetime. Your mom and dad will be around. Ryland and I will be fine."

"You know this makes you the cool wife, right?"

"Yeah," I tell him. "I know."

But when he takes off in August, Peg and Rand are also out of town, and Ryland and I are on our own. A week into Jeff's absence, when I'm nearing my wit's end with loneliness, I call one of my few friends who is also a mom—Brandy, an old college pal. She lives in San Jose with her husband and baby boy, Christopher, who arrived two months after Ryland did. "Fly down here with the baby and let's go to the beach," I tell her. "We need a mom's day out."

She makes arrangements to buzz down for the weekend to stay at my in-laws' weekend house on the boardwalk. We call around and invite a couple other girlfriends, and Macie—Jeff's longtime friend whom I've grown close with, and who is the only non-family member I leave Ryland with—offers to come along and babysit so that Brandy and I can relax. "You're welcome to host the girls at the beach house, but please be careful," Rand tells me when he calls to check in on us. "Remember what happened to those two girls not too long ago."

I remember. In October 2006, two girls from the University of San Diego and their boyfriends were staying at a condo near the boardwalk. In the middle of the night, three masked men found the front door unlocked, entered the house, forced the male victims into a bathroom at gunpoint, and gang-raped the two young women. Not only had it been all over the news for months, and not only were the defendants convicted and sentenced to life in prison in early 2008, but a family friend who was a detective told Jeff and Rand that it was the worst case of sexual assault that he'd seen in the history of his career. It was in a rougher part of Mission Beach, where a lot of college kids rent condos, and it was a good distance from Jeff's family's beach house. "I'll be careful," I promise Rand. "There will be a lot of us there, and we'll only be out in the daytime."

My childhood best friend Casey and five other girlfriends join us, and the only difference between this and the old days is that

Ryland, now eight months old, and six-month-old Christopher have joined us to supply even more laughs than ever. We spend the day lounging on the beach until the late afternoon, when we put on sundresses and open a bottle of wine to relax in the front room. Macie takes the babies upstairs and puts them to bed as the rest of us kick around the thought of going for a bike ride on the boardwalk. Brandy comes with me to the kitchen to prepare a few snacks, telling me about a sign language class in which she's just enrolled Christopher.

"Sign language?" I ask her. "He eats and he sleeps. What could he possibly need to tell you?"

"No, Hill, it's amazing. They learn the signs to tell you when they're hungry, or when their tummies are full," she says. "They learn 'mommy,' and 'daddy' . . . honestly, you should think about it."

Right then, I hear the front door open. Stretching my neck into the living room, I can't place who would just be entering. Peering around the kitchen doorway, I meet my girlfriends' faces—all blank, as if they're stifling some kind of panic. "What in the . . ." I step slowly into the room to join them, and find two men—wearing baggy shorts and white socks up to their knees, with shaved heads and tattoos—who have cruised through the front door and are standing in our living room. Their arms are crossed; they look me up and down, bold as can be.

The first thing that comes to my mind is the infamous attack of the USD students.

The second thing that comes to my mind: *Our babies are upstairs.*

My friends all sit frozen, their eyes planted on me in silent terror. My fight-or-flight response kicks in immediately.

I march toward the men and stick my finger in one of their faces. "My husband is upstairs, and he will *not* be happy if he comes down here right now!"

His stare moves from my mouth to my hand . . . where I see him take note that I'm wearing a wedding band. He squints his eyes, and stares me down. We stay this way for what feels like minutes—in reality, maybe a couple of breaths, if I were calm enough to breathe right now.

Slowly, he turns his face and looks toward his friend. *This is it,* I think. This is the pivotal moment: either they have weapons and they'll attack us, or they'll turn around and back out.

Now they're both staring at me, their lips puckered up tough. They exchange one more glance between themselves. In my peripheral vision I keep my attention on their hands, holding my breath, anchoring my leg to kick one of them in the groin and poke the other in the eye, just as Jeff has taught me.

Then, they both turn around and swagger out the front door. I slam it behind them. "Lock everything! Close all the blinds!"

My friends all scramble to secure every possible entryway while I dial 911. Within a few minutes, the police arrive. After they leave with full descriptions of the two men, we split the blinds open to find them being arrested on the boardwalk. Later, the police tell us that their excuse was that they'd mistaken our beach house for a bar, but they both end up in the back of police cars and in jail for the night with a public drunkenness charge.

As the police cars drive off, my friends are in awe. "I thought *I* was a protective mama bear!" Brandy says. The event proves—to me, even more than to any of them—the courage I possess when it comes to Ryland's well-being. I'm willing to put my own life in danger for my child, and in this moment, I embrace my new role in the world: I'm Ryland's protector, for as long as I live.

AFTER ANOTHER WEEK with little communication beyond the occasional email, Jeff returns safely from Indonesia. On hearing the story, he asks me to vow to stay closer to home, and I agree without hesitation.

Most mornings, I put Ryland in the stroller and walk to the supermarket to pick up groceries for dinner or to shop at one of the discount department stores that are located in the plaza a few blocks from our house. We're on a tight budget, so it's rare that I actually shop, but we visit so frequently that I learn what days of the week their new shipments arrive, so sometimes I pick up a cute new dress for my baby girl.

One afternoon, in the checkout line, Ryland sits calmly in the stroller when I spot the most adorable little bow fastened around the head of the baby in front of us. "I love her bow!" I tell the mother, and when she turns around, it's clear she's about my age.

"Oh, thank you!" she says. "Actually my sister makes these and sells them really cheap."

"It's so cute. Ryland, do you like the baby's bow?" Ryland stares at me with wide eyes, then bobs her head toward the baby.

"I'm going to see my sister next weekend," the mom says. "I'd be happy to get one for your little girl, if you like?"

We both pay in haste and shuffle toward the store's exit to exchange phone numbers. I realize that this woman—Jenn, as she introduces herself—and her husband live just a few minutes from Jeff and me. Similar to our situation, her husband works a lot, and Jenn craves having a buddy to get out with in the daytime.

The following week, we meet up. She hands me a bundle of hair bows in fabrics of polka dots and butterflies and my favorite of all, one that's leopard print and pink. "Gosh, I can't tell you how happy I am to meet another mom," I tell her.

"So am I," she says. "I need more friends around here with children!" We make a plan for later in the week to take our babies on a walk around nearby Lake Murray. Ryland and Jenn's baby, Gianna, are within a few weeks of each other's age, so Jenn and I keep each other in patient company when one of us needs to stop for a bench break to feed one of the babies. During these moments of quiet sharing, many of our conversations center around grief. Jenn lost her brother-in-law, with whom she and her husband were extremely close, right around the same time that my brother passed away. Like me, she's trying to balance taking full responsibility for another human being—Gianna—with the emotional side of herself, which still needs so much care. I understand this completely, and between us, there's a sense of belonging and togetherness. For the first time in a very long time, I don't feel lonely.

Our mornings out together also give me a confidence in my mothering that frees me up to stand back and enjoy watching Ryland learn and develop. Jenn inspires me—whereas I'm usually in capris and a ball cap, she always does her lipstick and slides on sunglasses, looking pulled together and complete. In college, she studied early childhood education and always has the latest news on what we should be feeding the girls and cool new techniques to stimulate their brains and overall development. I learn so much as we push our daughters along the hike-and-bike trail around Lake Murray, absorbing the sun and this, the pure satisfaction and indulgence of motherhood. Our girls clap and laugh and stretch their arms wide open toward all there is to take in around us: the ducks dipping their beaks into the lake in search of fish, the tall reeds swaying in the breeze, the prickly pear cactus plants dotting the surroundings with their bright red figs. Gianna is very vocal, constantly cooing and giggling and trying to engage Ryland's attention, while Ryland is quieter, like a little sponge with how she observes everything we pass. As she glances around in awe of the beautiful world she's found herself in, the sunlight beams on my little girl's shiny blond hair like a halo. "Ryland," I say, but I'm pleased when she is too caught up in wonder to crane her glance back toward me from the seat of her stroller. I know Jenn is thinking the same thought about Gianna that I'm thinking about Ryland: *I wish I could keep her this happy forever.*

After a couple of months, Jenn shares an idea that she's been pondering. "I'm thinking about signing Gianna up for baby sign language classes."

"It's so funny you say that," I tell her. "Right before I met you, one of my friends who lives up in San Jose told me she'd just signed her baby up for those."

"I took three years of ASL in college. They say that babies know what they want but don't have the verbal capacity to express it, and that really frustrates them—"

"They're infants!" I say with a laugh. "It's so funny to think they have any frustration in the world."

"You're telling me Ryland's never thrown a tantrum that you couldn't figure out the solution to?"

"Oh . . ."

"Exactly."

We learn that there's an up-and-coming baby boutique in

the notoriously hip area of North Park that's offering a Sunday morning free baby sign class for parents to sample and see if they like it enough to enroll.

On the Thursday before we're supposed to meet for the intro class, my in-laws offer to babysit Ryland to give me a day to get some things done. The timing of all this strikes me—alarms me—that Friday, two days before the class, when I get a phone call from my father-in-law. I've just clicked Ryland into her high chair for her lunch when the phone rings. I nestle the wireless receiver between my ear and my shoulder and answer. "Hello?"

"Hill," Rand says. "Can you talk?"

"Hi, Rand, yeah, of course. I'm just getting ready to feed the baby."

"That's actually why we're calling. Hill, uh . . ." Through the phone, he struggles. "Peg and I are concerned about the baby."

I glance at Ryland, who's secure in her high chair. Then, cautiously, I reach for a chair and slowly take a seat. "You're concerned? Why?"

"We really think her hearing needs to be checked."

I stay silent, trying to grasp any one of the emotions that are surging through me right now—panic, a mix of shame for what I fear was unintentional ignorance and negligence as a new parent on my part, a gratefulness that my in-laws care so much about my daughter, and a shame for my anger that their concern is about to turn our world upside down. He continues. "She isn't responding the way she should be to sounds."

I steady myself, my fear taking shape as a reality like a waterfall freezing midstream. A month ago, I called the pediatrician because I'd begun to wonder whether Ryland's behavior was normal. Loud noises never seemed to frighten her. She still wasn't answering to her own name. The nurse at the pediatrician's office offered to make an appointment for us, but I told her I'd look at my schedule and call her right back. Then, because Ryland is perfect and because to think that anything could be wrong with her was the most terrifying thought I could imagine . . . I talked myself out of going. I haven't called back since.

"We've been watching her, Hill," Rand says, "and this is something we've been noticing for a while now. We're worried. I think something needs to be done."

With the air knocked out of me, I manage to tell him, "I'll talk to Jeff, Rand. Thanks for letting me know."

That phone call is the final push that I need. I click the TALK button on the phone to turn it off, then turn it immediately back on. I dial our pediatrician's office. "Mrs. Whittington, hi," the nurse says. Immediately she hears the new urgency in my tone. "If I squeeze Ryland in for two o'clock today, can you come in?"

"Yes," I tell her. "We'll be there."

Ryland's face is confused as I rush around the house and load her into the car. On the way to the appointment, I begin to run scenarios in my head: I think of the signs that I've allowed to convince me that Ryland can hear . . . then all of the many signs that have made me worry maybe she can't. Jeff and I had taken note that the only toys she likes to play with are ones with mechanized motion or flashing lights—visual toys. Only when we tap her shoulder can we get her attention, and when she's upset, she doesn't calm to our voices unless she actually sees us enter the room.

I enter the pediatrician's office gripping Ryland in my arms. I'm usually excited for her to see the pediatrician, to get the news that she's in perfect health and here's what stages are coming next and here are the new foods that are age-appropriate for her to try now . . . but today, inside the waiting room, the cartoon animal décor and bright colors seem darker than they ever seemed before—and for the first time, I realize that the doctor's office is not a cheery place for every parent who comes in.

The pediatrician enters the exam room, smiling as usual. He's young, thin, and handsome, with young children of his own. "You always have the answers," I tell him. "We needed to come and see you today."

On the chair of the exam room, I sit Ryland down and reach in my diaper backpack to pull out the hand puppet that I always carry to keep her occupied. She takes it, balling up its fuzzy nose in her fist.

"Something isn't right with Ryland," I tell the doctor. "I seriously think . . ."

He listens patiently as I search for my words.

"I'm afraid I've been in denial." Right here, the fears that have been shoring up inside me bust open like a broken dam. "She isn't talking or turning toward sounds. I really think she may not be hearing. . . ."

"Mrs. Whittington, listen," he says. "Children develop at different stages, and Ryland could just be a late talker. If anything, maybe it's possible she could need ear tubes." I watch as he turns and types something into the laptop he carries, then turns to me. "I typically don't order hearing tests until children are eighteen months old, but I sense your concern, so I'll go ahead and order a BAER test."

"A BAER test?"

"It is a sedated hearing test that measures brain wave activity in response to certain sounds. I'll go ahead and send a request to your insurance company, but it could take a few weeks to get in, depending on when they have an appointment available. And Mrs. Whittington, really—I wouldn't lose any sleep over this," he says, "I'm sure she's just fine."

I leave the pediatrician's office and call Jeff, not at all appeased. Something inside me knows that I'm right: my daughter cannot hear. "'I wouldn't lose any sleep over it,' he says!" I tell Jeff. "Clearly he's not a mother!"

When we arrive home, I keep things quiet . . . not because I think noise will disturb Ryland from unwinding for her nap, but because there's a part of me now that doesn't want to leave her out of any sensory experiences that I can enjoy. I call my cousin Melissa, who offers to come stay the night with me. I accept immediately, knowing she will be a strong shoulder for me to cry on.

And then that night, almost as if she can sense my worry, Ryland decides to take her first steps.

I videotape her walking back and forth on our living room floor, both concentrating and smiling in her cow-print, fuzzy jumper. My feelings are mixed as I videotape: I'm beside myself with excitement for this new stage, but deep down, I know that normal stages of development like this one won't always come easily for this sweet little girl.

Melissa stands quietly with me when I put Ryland down for bed. We exit Ryland's room and stand just outside her doorway. "Let's stay here a minute until she falls asleep," I whisper. "I want to try something."

She nods in cooperation. "Okay."

When the room has gone completely silent, we exchange the glance of a shared mission: our eyes meet, I bite my lip, and I nod as I push open the door and we begin our tiptoe back into the nursery. I look at Melissa . . . and then I let out a loud whistle.

Nothing.

"Ryland!" I shout. "*Ryyyy*-land!"

Ryland doesn't even stir.

"Come with me," I tell Melissa. We march toward the kitchen and load our arms with pots and pans, a wooden spoon in my grip. We *clang, clang, clang* them together . . . and Ryland stays sleeping, soft and sound.

I haven't slept when Jeff returns home in the morning wearing his pressed navy blue uniform. Immediately, he hugs and kisses me. I begin to weep in his arms. "When she wakes up," he says, "I'll try it, too."

Comforted by his concern, I nod. After Ryland is awake and fed, we sit her in the middle of the family room floor so she can play. Jeff goes into her toy chest and picks up a couple of wooden blocks. He walks up behind Ryland and looks at me, pained by what he's about to do. Then he stretches both arms widely and smacks the blocks together.

The cracking sound echoes through our home—in fact, I flinch, knowing that if any of our neighbors were sleeping, they're definitely not now.

But Ryland doesn't budge. She remains contently focused on her toys.

Jeff knows as well as I do that we have a problem, and we're in need of some answers.

I PUT ON a big pot of coffee for both sets of grandparents before they show up. All four of them are solemn when they come through our door, but I can see that they're trying to be strong for us. As our baby girl walks across the room, back and forth, showing off the new skill she's mastered, our parents respond with big smiles and cheers. It's evident that each of us is grieving a future that we'd been imagining for Ryland . . . but I feel a certain comfort knowing that our parents are here to stand with us through this.

As my parents, in-laws, and husband enter the kitchen to have some coffee, I excuse myself to my bedroom upstairs. I close the door, slump into a seat on the bed, and, wailing, I let it all go: the fears, the pain, the hopes I'd had for my daughter. Will Ryland have a silent future? I picture her as a teenager, sitting with us at a family Thanksgiving celebration, where we're all laughing and listening to music. Will Ryland exist alone, in silence? And am I being overly dramatic? I've envisioned her future with that all-American scenario: married, with two kids, the house, and the white picket fence. It's never occurred to me that my version of Ryland's perfect life may be a little different from her reality.

The next day is the last Sunday of January 2009. When I wake up, I'm amazed that I was able to sleep, and I'm resolved and ready to move forward to the next step. Jeff has taken the day off of work to attend the first day of sign language class with us. He drives Jenn, Gianna, Ryland, and me on the twenty-five-minute trip to So Childish. "Oh, it's cute," muses Jenn when we find the quaint little shop that sits on the corner of a street that's known for its historical buildings. With plenty of spare time before the class begins, we browse the boutique—it features everything from the latest toys to sing-along music books with matching puppets to gorgeous brand-name clothes, some made from organic fabrics, and a pyramid that serves as the store's centerpiece, stacked high with luxe cloth diapers. "Wow," Jenn murmurs to me. "You'd have a field day if you were planning a baby shower."

A baby shower is the last thing on my mind right now.

We fold the girls' strollers and climb through the crowd of moms and babies—the trial class is jam-packed. It's the typical Southern California mix of moms: some very put together and pretty, in cute jackets and big earrings and heels; others minimalist and Californian, in yoga pants and long tunics or flowy skirts and sandals.

The room is turquoise, with painted murals of children playing. It's large enough to double as a play zone for babies to go when their moms are shopping and a class isn't being held, but the orange-cushioned benches that line the room provide a stashing place for all the toys. The room has soft carpet and a barn-style half door to separate the classroom from the boutique, so children are viewable but contained. Our girls take it all in, jibber-jabbering with each other, as Jenn makes polite conversation with the moms sitting near us. One tells Jenn that she's come just because she's dying to meet other mothers. I overhear another brag that her eight-month-old is already pulling herself up by the edge of the couch and trying to take a step. Jenn leans in to me. "You're quiet," she says. "You okay?"

"Yeah," I say with a nod, shaking off her concern. But my purpose for being here isn't quite like the other moms'. The signs I've been overlooking creep back into my mind for the thousandth time in the past two days. How had I not known that my little girl couldn't hear? Ryland is so healthy, happy, and typical to her peers, I've believed . . .

That is, until we met Jenn and Gianna. As I've seen how alert and verbally responsive Gianna is, a concern began to rise in me. I'd begun to question why Ryland isn't learning to say "momma" or "dada" like Gianna mastered months ago. Who really ever thinks their child has something "wrong" with them? Have I been living in denial?

There's a collective straightening up among all of us moms, as Monta, the baby sign teacher, emerges at the front of the room. She's written a bestselling book on baby sign language and is known as one of the pioneers of this field. As Monta introduces herself, I find myself relaxing into her presence—she's in her mid-thirties, a natural beauty with short brown hair and a gorgeous smile. She's cheerful and animated with the children, and next to her sits a stuffed teddy bear. After she goes through some of the basics about the class, she sits down on a stool and pulls the bear onto her lap. Jenn and I are as amazed as the children are when Monta slips on a pair of white gloves and slides her arms inside the bear's arms. When Monta begins to speak by using her hands, it actually appears that the bear is the one doing the signing! "Anybody up for some music?" she says. She hits the button on a music player and begins to sign the words to a children's song.

"Ryland," I tell her. "Music!"

"Clap, Ryland," Jeff urges.

Ryland watches Monta intently but appears more spellbound by the motion of her signing than by the actual song itself. The other babies in the room smile up at their mothers, shrill their voices in thrill, bounce to the music, and flag their arms with the sound . . . all of them, that is, except for Ryland. Our little girl does nothing to respond to the music; it's as if she's in her own little world. The truth is beginning to crystallize. Ryland cannot hear. In this communal setting, the even heavier thought occurs to me: my daughter is left out of experiencing life as the other babies are.

Suddenly, it makes sense that she loves her fire truck toy so much—the noise is enough to make me crazy, but she loves how visual it is, with its relentless flashing light. I also remember a trip we'd taken a couple of months ago to Maui to visit Jeff's brother Jay. We were relaxing on the patio when their other brother, Scott, came out and said, "Have you guys had Ryland's hearing checked?"

As we followed him inside toward the room where she was sleeping, he explained that he'd heard Ryland waking up in her crib, and when he went in the room and called her name, she didn't turn toward him.

We followed him into her room, but we didn't really think much of it at the time—we appreciated Scott's concern, but he was her uncle! To us it was just sort of cute for him to fuss about her. When the three of us entered and found her in her crib, she was sitting up, smiling. When Scott approached her to pick her up out of her bed, she started waving her hands in circles. "See?" Jeff said. "She's okay."

We didn't know enough then to acknowledge the truth that's now growing clearer.

After class, Jenn continues in her friendly exchanges with other mothers. Jeff engages with Ryland and Gianna, kicking inside their strollers, while I approach Monta in the only quiet corner in the room. "Can I talk to you?"

"Sure." I'm soothed, at least a little, by her warmth.

"Um . . ." I wring my hands. I feel as though sharing this with another person is about to make it all true . . . but I have to look out for Ryland. "I feel like maybe I was meant to come here today," I tell her, trying to control an unsteadiness in my throat. "I'm not positive, but I've been getting some clues that my little girl can't hear."

"Clues?"

"She's not speaking, she doesn't turn to us when we say her name, she didn't really seem all that interested in the sound of the songs you were playing. . . ." I look at her with desperation, not wanting to list any more of the signs—the many obvious signs.

Monta responds assuredly. "I know this is hard, but try to stay positive," she says. "Until you can speak with an audiologist, I'll do everything I can to help you."

She guides me to a bookshelf and fills me in on some resources, and alone, I make my way to the cash register. "Whatcha got there?" Jenn says. We both glance down to the stack of books in my arms: six copies of Monta's book. "I need to start studying," I whisper to her.

"Me, too, I'm rusty after all these years. I haven't used ASL since college!"

"No," I tell her. "Jenn . . . I really think Ryland is deaf."

"Hillary . . ." she says. "What makes you say that?"

"You've seen her," I say, tears welling in my eyes. "Gianna always responds to you; she can hear you. Ryland doesn't really respond to loud noises like she should. . . . I don't even know if she knows her name."

"Let's sign up for the class," she says. "When we get home, I'll help you get a jump start on some information and resources."

I SPEND ALL night in bed miming the signs in Monta's book. "Babe," Jeff says. "Please let's try not to jump to any premature conclusions with this until we know more." Jeff is so much more used to handling distress in a cool, collected way than I am.

"And who knows when that could be?"

"Let's just sleep on it tonight, okay? Tomorrow will be the start of the week. I'll call first thing and make an appointment at Children's Hospital."

When he follows through, I'm relieved to see that we're sharing the same grasp of the magnitude of what's happening. He wakes up earlier than usual, and when I bring coffee to him at the computer, I find that he's emailing his friend who's in medical school. "What are you saying to him?" I ask.

"I want to know if there are causes of hearing loss that are treatable or curable."

Then, at exactly eight o'clock, he calls a children's hospital in San Diego, whose audiologist's office says the earliest they could test Ryland would be in mid-March. Almost as if in response, we drive to Peg and Rand's. They assure us they have some friends around the city who might be able to at least recommend hearing specialists for us to see in the meantime. Peg accepts a handful of the copies of Monta's book that I've bought and pledges to pass them around our extended family. In my desperation, I'm buoyed by the sense of strength my in-laws are giving us: *We're all in this together.*

But late that night, I see for myself how upset my mother-in-law truly is when she accidentally copies me in on an email to a friend who's the president of the auxiliary for the children's hospital in San Diego. "We are really frustrated right now with what is going on with our grand-daughter, Ryland," she writes. "She is not hearing. She is also going to be 14 months old and she hasn't made any attempt to talk or make consonant sounds."

In the email, I pick out phrases like *beside ourselves with worry* and *our family is in such a state of unrest*. She continues: "Does my 20 years of supporting Children's Hospital give me any sort of edge to get this testing done sooner? Do you have any pull?"

There's nothing overtly offensive in the email, but something about it makes me feel guilty. The urgency of her request causes me to beat up on myself even more: how have we not seen the signs up to now? I've tried to be such a "hands-on" mother. I've stayed at home so that I can do everything to take care of her: I breastfed her, prepare homemade baby food, I sit on the carpet and play with her for hours. We're so involved in her life, yet we feel as though we've failed her in this moment in a way that may be irreversible. After I let Peg's email settle in, I make a decision never to let something like this happen again.

I also realize, quickly, that if I'm going to be strong enough to see Ryland through whatever's ahead, then I have to start to control my emotions and stop taking things personally—now. Ultimately, Peg's plea—along with our consistent phone calls to the audiology department every morning to see whether they've had any new cancellations—is successful. We're able to secure an appointment with an audiologist at the children's hospital in the first week of February. I am pure anxiety—both nervous and excited, just to get to the bottom of it . . . to know for certain whether there's an issue, so that we can set up a plan of action.

In the meantime, Jenn and I arrive early at So Childish to secure a spot in the front of the classroom. After a couple of weeks, I've learned everything I possibly can . . . but Ryland is more than a year old, and I know from what Jenn and I have chatted about that it's necessary to work constantly to increase a child's capacity for language. Very soon, she could need more signs than "eat," "milk," and "daddy." If there's a chance that Ryland's primary language is going to be sign, then I need to begin to learn to speak it—and teach it, to her and the whole family—fluently.

In need of something more advanced, I sign up for night classes taking American Sign Language at the local junior college. My brother-in-law Scott signs up with me, and since Jeff is working more often than not, Peg offers to watch Ryland on the nights we have class. She also manages to learn the entire baby sign language book before anyone else does, including me. It warms my heart to witness her incredible dedication to Ryland's future.

Every time Scott shows up, he signs *Hello*—a simple forehead-salute of the hand—which drives Ryland wild with laughter. One night, when he steps into the kitchen, she raises both hands and makes fast circles in the air, calling out.

"What is it, Ryland?" I ask her, both using my facial expression and the sign.

Again, she raises both hands and draws wild circles. When Scott comes back into the room, she stops the sign, giggles, and makes it again. I mimic the sign. "That's your uncle Scott!" She does it again, then goes crazy with claps and laughs. Then Scott makes the sign, and again, Ryland laughs like I've never heard her laugh before. Both awestruck, Scott and I exchange a glance, until I can muster the words: "I think that's her sign for Uncle Scott!"

Both to practice communicating with my little girl and to keep myself busy, in the days leading up to Ryland's appointment with the audiologist I work intensively at home to teach her sign. During these sessions, she is sometimes frustrated and aggressive toward my intent to teach her so much so quickly, is almost visibly resentful that we have to do this at all, but when she doesn't have my full attention, she is extremely clingy. All of it makes my heart cave in, time after time, and I learn to take moments in these days when we stop everything. I pick her up, and we sit on the couch or the mint green baby glider in her nursery, and I hold her. I caress her hair. Even if she can't hear my words, I tell her: "It's okay." I hum "Jesus Loves Me" like my mom used to sing to me when I was little, while I press her open palm to my throat and squeeze her little body against my chest. She seems to melt into the vibration of my voice coming through my throat and chest, and, even if just for a minute, I know that she understands that she is loved. I remind myself often that while my intention is to get her ready for her life, what Ryland needs most of all is her mommy's love.

One night, Jeff cleans up after dinner while I put Ryland down. Then we meet in the living room and begin to research what our options could possibly be if indeed Ryland is deaf. On YouTube, we stumble on a slew of videos of deaf children hearing for the first time after having had a procedure done to make it possible for them to hear. We both watch, our eyes glassy with tears, as the infants and toddlers and school-aged children and even one teen hear their parents' voices for the first time, or the sound of nurses clapping their hands and singing the children's names, or the click-clack tumble of Legos falling on a wooden desk inside the doctor's office. Some of the smaller children don't react at all, as if perhaps things were more peaceful in their minds before they were exposed to sound. Others call out or clap in sheer excitement, a new world having just opened to them.

Jeff and I sit, shoulder to shoulder, silent tears streaming down our faces. I have so many questions about cochlear implants zipping around my mind—Where is the best place in our area to have them done? Can any deaf child receive them? How much could they possibly cost, and would we ever be able to afford them? But the answer to one question is clear, just from the expression on my husband's face: we both want to give Ryland the chance to hear.

The second week in February, Jeff and I drive Ryland to her official hearing test—the BAER (brainstem auditory evoked response) test. For this test, Ryland needs to be sleep- and food-deprived so that they can sedate her safely and quickly. The only appointment we could get isn't until the afternoon, so we spend the morning being very creative to keep Ryland awake until it's time to leave for the hospital. We also head to Chuck E. Cheese to provide her with plenty of stimulation with the games and robotic puppet shows so that she'll stay happy until the appointment, but ready to zonk out when it's time for the test.

It's just Jeff and me in the exam room when the audiologist enters. She's friendly enough but focused on her task. She administers a sleep aid and waits for Ryland to fall asleep completely before she places electrodes on Ryland's scalp and then to each earlobe. With her back to us and with Ryland sleeping peacefully on the hospital bed, she begins to run the hearing test on Ryland. "It will take a little over an hour for the machine to monitor Ryland's neurological brain responses," she says. "I'll step out, but of course you can stay with her."

At this point, Jeff and I have already accepted the worst. Even without the diagnosis, we know that Ryland is deaf. We've already grieved the reality of our situation, and we've spent countless hours researching cochlear implants and the overwhelming number of steps necessary to obtain them. All we want now is the "official" news so that we can move forward with the time-sensitive process.

When the test is complete, the audiologist reenters. She's quiet, she folds her hands, she seems tense. "The test results show that Ryland isn't hearing anything except sounds at the top end of the spectrum," she says.

We sit calmly, and listen to her continue.

She looks at the ground and then squarely at us. "She is what we would consider to be profoundly deaf," she says.

Looking back, our lack of tears or emotion was probably a shock to the audiologist. Inside both of us was a strange comfort in the confirmation of what we already knew to be true.

"Right away we'll refer you to a pediatric ear, nose, and throat specialist. If there's any good news in this, due to the level of Ryland's hearing loss, it's safe to say she would be a candidate for cochlear implants," she says, "as long as she has the physical anatomy to receive them."

"Determined through a CAT scan . . . right?"

"That's correct. A CAT scan will confirm this."

CAT scan. I picture my baby asleep inside one of those horizontal, claustrophobic machines while a computer scans her brain. It's an unsettling thought, but I know it's one of the many necessary steps that we need to take.

As soon as we return home, Jeff and I continue with our research. A prevailing issue among parents with deaf children who have shared their experiences online is that their children who have received cochlear implants are often cast out of the Deaf community (who capitalize the letter *D* as part of their group identity). Some members of the community say that if a child can hear now, even if they were born deaf, then they simply don't belong. Everything about this experience is emotional enough, and the last thing I want is for my innocent little girl to gain hearing only to learn that she has instant enemies in the community whose language was once her only hope to communicate. I know that if I'm going to get through it in one piece, I'm going to need to surround myself with support. When I share this with Jeff, he immediately agrees that it would be helpful to reach out to other parents who might be able to share some wisdom.

"We don't want to allow our egos to get in the way," he says, acknowledging that we can't and won't ever know everything.

In the times that we've turned to parents and friends for a little guidance, we've learned that people who have experienced similar challenges before can provide some of the most important lessons we need. We've used our own judgment and life experiences to help us make the best decision possible for Ryland, but now it's time for us to allow ourselves to be vulnerable— even to strangers who might understand our situation better than we do.

Within a week of receiving Ryland's diagnosis, I locate a mom named Susan who used to head the support group in San Diego for families of children who have undergone cochlear implant surgery. I send her an email, asking her if we can plan to meet sometime. "It would be awesome to speak to some other families with hard of hearing children for support," I write to her. "We think it would really help us through this."

Susan responds, saying that her three-and-a-half-year-old son was diagnosed through his newborn hearing screening, "so we knew he was deaf right away," she says, sharing that when he was six months old, he was implanted bilaterally simultaneously (from my research, I know that this means in both ears, at the same time). "He hears and speaks beautifully," she says, "very instinctively and naturally. There is hope."

There is hope.

The busier I get, the more energy I find to get everything done. I start a binder to begin to keep track of all the doctors' appointments and meetings with organizations that friends of friends have been recommending for us. Within a few weeks, Ryland has a CAT scan completed, and the news is uplifting: Ryland continues to be candidate for cochlear implants.

First, she's fitted with hearing aids, which she'll wear for three months—a requirement from our insurance company, based upon Food and Drug Administration recommendations, to prove that a child doesn't benefit from the hearing aids and thus needs an invasive surgery like cochlear implants.

I learn the instructions (and the tricks) to care for the hearing devices. Every day, I test the batteries and clean the devices with alcohol swabs. I also take them off Ryland before we drive in the car. Otherwise, I'm forced to pull the car over when I hear the high-pitched screeching sound of hearing aid feedback as I look back to see Ryland sucking and chewing on one of the aids.

To add to the chaos in the short term but to aid with it in the long term, Jeff and I make an offer on a house—a bright, spacious, three-bedroom ranch with a sprawling front yard—that's just a couple of minutes from his parents' place so that they can be closer to help with the baby.

In spite of the diagnosis, throughout March things fall into place as smoothly as we could possibly ask, except for the most critical detail, which is to secure a date for Ryland's surgery. Every expert we've seen has told us that time is of the essence in implanting children with these cochlear devices, simply because after a certain stage in their toddler years, they can lose the ability to learn verbal language so that they can speak it normally. With each day she is missing the most critical childhood developmental stages in relation to hearing, speech and language, and communication; also, the area of the brain responsible for hearing, along with the auditory nerve, has gone an extensive period of time without the beneficial stimulation that allows the brain to evolve and change and become less responsive to any sound in the future.

This, of course, spurs my worry and makes me all the more anxious to schedule Ryland's surgery. With the hope of expressing the seriousness of our intention, we decide that Jeff will address it with the pediatric ear surgeon who heads the hearing and cochlear implant program at the children's hospital. In early April, he emails her. "We were given an anticipated date of some time in July for the procedure," my husband writes, "which seems much too far away for my family and me. My question for you is, can we get the surgery date scheduled now to avoid any delays, with the possibility for Ryland to be implanted in June? If the delay is for insurance reasons, then if necessary, I will be on the phone with them every day to make sure the approval process moves along."

Indeed it was an insurance issue, the doctor replies in a kind-toned email, but she agrees to set a date for May 28—the end of the month, but much better than July—so that things move along somewhat quickly when our insurance is approved. In the meantime, we do everything we can to push it all forward: Ryland is able to sign more than two hundred words, which will come in handy even after her surgery as she learns to speak. A large part of my days during this period is spent sitting on the gridlocked Southern California freeways, traveling from preoperation appointments to a speech therapist to meetings with allergists who are trying to solve a problem with Ryland's middle ear pressure that the ear, nose, and throat specialist has discovered, while I also try to get things organized for our move. During these drives, I call Jeff—sometimes as I'm wiping away my tears. "We're doing everything we can for her, Hill," he says. "We have to stay strong."

Ryland is such a trouper on these days that I always reward her with a Chicken McNuggets Happy Meal. The same question always comes through the drive-through speaker. "Is the Happy Meal for a girl or a boy?"

"It's for a girl."

I always unwrap the toy from the plastic and hand it back toward Ryland, bouncing and twirling the plastic Hello Kitty figurine or the Littlest Pet Shop animals under their pastel salon hair dryers. *No.* Ryland takes the toy in her hand and promptly throws it back at me. I cannot figure it out—is it because she wants a toy that's more visually engaging, with flashing and motion? One afternoon in the first week of May 2009—after I've just found out that Ryland's surgery on May 28 has been rescheduled until late July, because our insurance company insists on adhering to the three months hearing aid trial that the FDA recommends—I'm about to lose it. Fed up, I sign furiously to Ryland: "What is wrong?!"

She stares at me. In the silence between us, my heart softens at the awareness we seem to share: our situation is just not easy.

By late May, we're moved into the new house, where Ryland and Kobe love all the space to play and run. As much as we love our new home, Jeff and I are becoming increasingly frustrated and angered by our insurance company's decision to delay Ryland's surgery. We vow to do what we do best: fight for our child.

Despite our surgeon's caution that it would be a first for her to see an insurance company agree to shorten the three-month time frame, Jeff decides to take them head-on. He drafts up a letter and provides factual evidence that our child will never benefit from hearing aids. He makes it clear that delaying the surgery has the potential to do more harm than good.

Within two weeks, we receive the news that the insurance company has agreed to shorten the time frame. We're elated—we've won! Our surgeon is floored.

While we've gained only a few weeks' time, this is a monumental victory for our family, and proof that at times we'll need to challenge the medical providers to ensure that our child is taken care of. Finally, one more detail has been settled: Ryland's surgery is rescheduled for July 1.

One night after Ryland has gone to bed, I send out an email to all of our friends and loved ones to update them on the move, Ryland's surgery date, and the progress we're all making as we learn American Sign Language. One response to the email happens to be my favorite—it's from Monta, who says: "It sounds like things are really moving ahead, and I'm happy to be on your mailing list! Hillary, if you would ever be interested in teaching classes for me someday, let me know. You will be especially qualified to teach other parents to sign!"

She signs off with a smiley face, and for the first time, it occurs to me that maybe all this pain and struggle will bring me to help other families one day.

WE PREP FOR the July 1 procedure with an overwhelming number of appointments and tests. In the weeks leading up to the surgery, we're so intent to keep Ryland healthy that we quarantine her from other children. Two days before the procedure, probably because of stress, it's me, and not Ryland, who gets sick with a cold.

Out of worry for Ryland, we send her to Jeff's parents' house. *This wasn't the plan,* I think to myself. Being without her makes my heart ache so deeply, but I know I have to protect her, even if that means we have to be apart.

When the morning of the procedure arrives, Jeff and I wake before dawn with my parents and drive to pick up Ryland down the street at Peg and Rand's. We videotape the trip to the hospital. I sit in the backseat of the car between my mom and Ryland, who's smiling and giggling. She has no idea that this will be the hardest day of her life, and therefore, of mine and Jeff's, too: this procedure will take six hours, though the doctors have told us to prepare to be at the hospital for as long as twelve.

Ryland's cooperation as we're putting her into her gown crushes me even more. She looks to me in confusion as the anesthesiologist prepares to sedate her with a mask that releases an anesthetic combined with fruit flavoring for patients who are children. *I love you, Ry,* I sign to her, fighting my tears. Right after Ryland is asleep, we walk alongside her as they wheel our baby girl through the hospital corridor toward the operating room.

On the way, we pass through a section of the hospital with an entryway marked PEDIATRIC ONCOLOGY UNIT. "You know what, Hill?" Jeff says, an optimistic calm suddenly filling his voice.

I look up at him.

"I just realized: this could be *so* much worse."

I take his hand. I think of the families who have occupied the rooms inside this hallway, how all of them would probably trade places with us in a heartbeat.

Chapter Three

The Gift of Sound

After six hours punctuated by just a few updates, the surgeon emerges from the operating room. She's smiling. "Good news," she says. "We'll be releasing Ryland to come home with you tonight."

"So it all went perfectly?" Jeff asks.

"*Perfectly*," she says.

Jeff and I grip each other's hands in relief as the staff wheels our little one, still sleepy, a little confused, and now wearing a white gauze bandage that's wrapped securely about the circumference of her tiny head, into the recovery room to come fully out of anesthesia. Here the surgeon briefs us on the details. "As you know," she says, "what we implanted today were the internal units that will process sound signals for Ryland's brain to receive." We were well aware of this part and had studied about it thoroughly: part of the implant surgery required them to drill into Ryland's skull to secure these internal units so that they sit flush with the head. "I took my time and implanted these very precisely," the doctor says, "so that even with a ponytail, Ryland's external processors will hang symmetrically."

For our child to come through this surgery was the greatest concern, but now, knowing that the doctor did what she could to make the implants *look* as normal as possible, Jeff and I clench our hands tighter together. *It's all going to be okay.* Throughout our research, as we've seen images of cochlear implants, a good way to describe them is that they look like an oversize hearing aid. The bulk of the implant is the sound processor and the battery that sits behind the ear, with a hook that goes over the ear to keep it in place. Coming off the implant is a wire that's two and a half inches long and connects to a round, quarter-sized disk, called the headpiece. The headpiece is held in place by a magnet that is implanted under the skin, and sits on the side of the head, behind and above the ear.

"It will take three to six weeks for the incisions to heal," the doctor continues, "and at that stage, we'll fit Ryland with the external processors that will transmit the sound to her brain."

"And then will come the day we've all been waiting for!" Jeff says excitedly

"That's right," says the surgeon. "Activation day."

Activation day is a well-known milestone among families of cochlear implant patients. That's the event that we've watched strangers celebrate in YouTube videos; it's the moment we've discussed with Susan and Monta and the families whose children also have had cochlear implants.

It's also the day that will determine whether the implants have worked. Our research has informed us about the troubling aspect of cochlear implants: they aren't guaranteed to be successful. The doctors have told us that many implanted children don't learn to speak, and their eventual hearing is less than marginal. But the success stories lift our hopes, showing us how possible it is that Ryland will be able to communicate with her peers, listen to music, and appreciate all the sounds in our environment that Jeff and I hear every day without even giving it a second thought.

The next morning, we surprise Ryland with a dollhouse when she wakes up, and we give her Popsicles and Jell-O whenever she asks. But her eyes have swollen shut from the invasiveness of the surgery, which makes our hearts ache even harder. Per the doctor's instructions, for the first seven days we keep the incisions completely dry. We never leave her side—we even sleep on the couch in the living room beside her.

Our main goal is to keep Ryland happy and keep her mind off the pain as much as we possibly can, but even to look at the incisions is intense. I can't imagine what they must feel like for a twenty-month-old. We take her for rides around our yard in her wagon, and we try everything we can think of to make her laugh. Every time a gentle smile breaks on her sweet face, we know that we are all making progress.

One point that we can't seem to agree on is our family's use of sign language. Jeff believes it would be best to wean Ryland off sign right away so that she'll be eager to learn verbal language as soon as she's able, but I don't want Ryland to find herself in a world that's completely new, suddenly unable to express herself or to understand us. For these few weeks, we decide, we'll use signs until she learns to speak.

At Ryland's three-week checkup, it's more good news: the incisions have healed, and the audiologists can program Ryland's devices. The morning that she'll be activated, I dress her in one of my favorite toddler outfits with the intent to capture the momentous events on camera: a pink-and-black polka-dot top with matching bloomers and black satin Mary Janes with a pink flower on the side. I do her hair, as usual, and put in a matching bow.

One fortunate thing about the future, I figure, is that Ryland is a girl and can keep her hair long over her processors, if she chooses that.

Our drive to the hospital is quiet, the air between Jeff and me tense with a combination of excitement and fear that I couldn't have even anticipated. From the waiting room, the pediatric audiology nurse invites us into the audiologist's office, and the experience inside is heightened by even more anxiety, though I figure that if I'm hiding mine from Ryland as well as Jeff is, then we're still doing okay.

Jeff stands, prepared to shoot video to capture the magical moment in the same way we've watched dozens of other parents do. I take a seat with Ryland, who seems to sense something big is happening, on my lap. The audiologist fidgets with a mechanical device and then turns to us. "Ready?"

I lean in and say softly to Ry: "Are you ready, Ry?" Ryland is tentative, slightly clinging to me. Jeff and I exchange a glance, and then Jeff tells her: "I think we're ready." I try to brace myself for what's coming next, with no idea what it might be: laughter? Surprise? Screams? Tears?

The audiologist turns a knob on her machine, then immediately begins to clap her hands—loudly. With the intensity of her clapping and the acoustics in the room, each clap is like a crack of lightning in my ears.

Ryland's body freezes. For these first couple of seconds, my mind races to translate what it means. Then, in a slow but desperate motion she grabs for me, grasps on to me, buries her head into my neck.

"Oh, sweetie," I tell her, not knowing what to do: instantly, it's clear that she is not a fan of the new sensation. I look to the audiologist with question in my eyes, hoping she will get the message. Do I ask her to stop clapping, or do we endure the discomfort of newness in hopes that Ryland will adjust? She continues to clap in a way that honestly might threaten to puncture even my ears. I expected us to use our voices, or maybe music—anything but *this* as the first sound our child would hear. I doubt this is a video we'll ever post on YouTube.

We arrive at home, and this time I take the video camera as Jeff opens the car to pull Ryland out. As he unbuckles her car seat, now in more familiar territory, she seems more comfortable, more curious. In the driveway, Jeff holds her against him in the open, in the sunshine of day. Here Ryland's eyes rise quickly to the sky.

"What does she hear?" I ask out loud, and then Jeff calls it.

"That's an airplane!"

She points up to the sky and then smiles at Jeff, double-checking to make sure that he hears it, too. She picked up on the sound even before we did.

Kobe exits the garage and bounces into the driveway to join us, barking and coaxing Ryland in a way that's almost comically ceremonial, as if he too is aware that something's changed since this morning. Ryland looks at Jeff and smiles, as if to say, "That's our dog, Daddy!" She's realizing that today, her relationship with everything and everyone in her world is new. She clasps her hand around her ear, as though she's trying to touch the sound itself.

There is an instant difference in our awareness of Ryland's

presence in our home and family—she learns her name quickly and answers to it by raising her eyes to us even from across the room. We enroll her in a special needs preschool class, and she's going on more playdates and is more engaged with her friends like Gianna, as well as her toys (though the ones that kick and zoom and flash still seem to attract her the most, which makes sense to Jeff and me since her deafness caused her to become a visual learner). She's also more alert and involved in the fun and laughter at family gatherings, and no parent has ever been as pleased to hear their child say, "I have big booger!" than I am when Ryland constructs a full sentence to announce this to me.

After the first few weeks, however, we note that not all aspects of her adaptation seem to come so easily. There are ongoing red flags, like her refusal to wear her "ears" and the fact that every time she hears a loud noise her eyes blink very hard in reaction. It is heartbreaking, and as the weeks go on, Jeff and I are dissatisfied with the responses we're receiving from her medical providers.

"She just needs to keep wearing them," they tell us. "She'll adjust."

Eventually, we've had enough. We agree that it's time to seek out an expert whose approach is as sensitive as a child in this situation needs, and we finally secure an appointment with Joan Hewitt, a world-class pediatric audiologist in San Diego. Our insurance won't cover it, but we can't take another day of seeing Ryland in such obvious discomfort.

Through her evaluation, Dr. Hewitt determines that Ryland's devices have been turned up far too loudly, which is why the sounds she experienced on activation day were so incredibly harsh for her. We learn that excessive eye-blinking is an uncontrollable reflexory response to loud noises when the implants are turned up too high. As relieved as we are to find a source of the problems we had identified, once again Jeff and I find ourselves sitting in frustration and guilt with the knowledge that Ryland has been having these unpleasant experiences since her activation day.

Joan continues her work and soon presents us with one of the biggest gifts Jeff could ever dream for. Ryland's been referring to him as "Wawa," something that our previous providers told us was normal. Upon hearing this, Joan makes a few adjustments to Ryland's program, and within seconds, she turns to Ryland. "Ryland," Dr. Hewitt says. "Say *Dada*."

"Dada."

Jeff looks at me with wide eyes that are quickly welling up, his heart clearly melting. We're decided: we will incur any expense necessary to be sure that Ryland receives the best care possible.

In early December 2009, we throw a second birthday party for her at Chuck E. Cheese. Macie joins us to help manage the scene with more than a dozen kids packed into our party space of two tables, one with a high chair for Miss Ryland at the head. Jenn hand sews a long-sleeved shirt, with the number 2 in a bold and blazing leopard-print pink pattern, paired with a handmade black-and-pink tutu and matching hair bows. (I realize only after we've arrived that I, too, have dressed in pink and black.) Ryland's cochlear implants are colored the same flesh tone as her skin, and they're so much a part of her now that only occasionally does it dawn on me that she's wearing them. To me this party feels like even more than a birthday celebration. It's Ryland's official coming-out to show us all that she's here to experience life just like every other kid does.

Our little guests can barely sit still long enough to get through lunch, and we load them each with tokens to go wild at the arcade games. I snap a photo of Rand helping Ryland to point a gun at an alien-hunting game, and another of Ryland "driving" Gianna inside a red convertible mechanical car. After lunch, I set down a cake decorated with a smiling sunshine and pastel flowers. Jeff holds Ryland and helps her to blow out the candles—of course it is he, Superdad and fire hero, who blows out the flame in the end.

On the ride home, in the passenger seat I spin around for a peek at her. In her car seat, she's surrounded on both sides by gifts wrapped and tied in a bow in every shade of pink. Looking peaceful, her head is tilted completely to one shoulder—she's fast asleep, with a pink binky in her mouth. I pull the camera back out of my purse and snap a photo. I have to remember this day that left my baby so blissfully exhausted.

Chapter Four

Clothing Catastrophes

We revel over the Christmas holidays, too, when Ryland can fully participate in her role as the center of everyone's attention, but into the new year in 2010, the parenting challenges continue. I might embrace them more easily if I could be sure that they were the normal speed bumps of toddler development, but Jeff and I agree that something remains a little off.

We enroll Ryland in a school for the deaf and hard of hearing so that she can get a foundation for learning some of the basics that might serve her before kindergarten. I also love the idea of exposing her to other deaf and hard of hearing children, with and without cochlear implants, so that she can feel understood among a group of children and families who will be sympathetic to our struggles. In this school, we agree with the administrators that she should be placed in the verbal communication class in hopes she will learn to rely on sound rather than signs. It comforts me to know that the teacher is fluent in ASL, in case there is a communication breakdown.

At home, I work on Ryland's speech and hearing around the clock, and Ryland's speech therapist, Gwen, evaluates her speech production development each week. Gwen gives me a list of homework assignments that consist of various speech exercises, activities, and role-playing, and of reading Ryland a minimum of ten books a day. Gwen also gives me a folder with different articles and advice on how to achieve the best hearing environments. She says that if we work hard and help Ryland continue to communicate, we could possibly mainstream her into regular school by kindergarten. Jeff and I agree that we want her to go to the school in our neighborhood—the same elementary school that he attended—with all of the neighbor kids. It's close to our home, safe, and rated among the best in our district. This is our goal, but we always keep it in perspective: it may not be possible.

Throughout every single day, I use speech exercises with Ryland—sometimes without her even realizing that I'm trying to teach her. We use flash cards with a reward system, hide plastic farm animals in boxes, make puppets and games . . . you name it, we do it. I feel like I'm under the gun to catch Ryland up to speed, especially because I still feel so guilty for the delay of her diagnosis. I have to make up for two years of lost hearing time. I've been around enough deaf and hard of hearing children to know that every one of them has different factors affecting their speech and hearing development, their success, and their school placement. Jeff and I want to make sure we do everything in our power to give Ryland the tools she needs. When she's unable to conquer a certain sound or activity after the first few tries, I beat myself up with the fear that I'm not doing enough for her.

But I never give up. I take Ryland on outings all over San Diego—to the park, to the zoo, the beach, the famous San Diego County Fair, held in Del Mar—anywhere that I think might stimulate her curiosity to communicate and learn. I talk to Ryland every opportunity that I can, even when the conversation seems meaningless: "Mommy is combing her hair, brushing her teeth, and putting her shoes on." She humors these efforts by granting me at least a couple of seconds of her attention, which, bless her, is usually enough to satisfy me with the knowledge that she's absorbing language.

As time progresses, Jeff and I are ecstatic that her verbal skills are beginning to explode. We begin to limit her sign language usage to certain activities like bathing, swimming, and early mornings, before we've put on her implants and she's too sleepy to want to talk.

With Ryland gone at school every morning, I sometimes feel like I'm on a deserted island. Because there are postoperation costs like speech therapy that we have to pay out of pocket, Jeff is held up working more than ever.

With no one to talk to who can understand us, I'm at a loss for how to deal with two issues that Ryland's still having: the first is that she's wetting the bed every night—and sometimes herself multiple times a day, which is something we had been trying to train her out of since right around her second birthday, shortly after she had the cochlear implants put in. Her school is a diaper-free zone, and the classroom has a restroom attached directly to it, but it doesn't seem to matter. I have no choice but to send Ryland to school with extra clothes every day; I figure maybe I screwed up by trying to potty-train her too early after the implants—maybe it was just too much change for her all at once—but part of me believes it's deeper than that. No matter how many times we try to explain to her that it's important for her to tell us or her teacher when she needs to go potty, it's the one thing she can't seem to catch on to and that continues to confound us.

Also, even after months have passed and Ryland is growing so well adjusted to most every other aspect of life with sound, there's a tantrum I face anytime I'm trying to get her out the door: she refuses to wear the clothes that I pick out.

It's not even that she wants to have a say in the choice or some kind of collaborative role; it's that she *hates* her clothes. Her dresses, her sweaters, the shoes I used to put on her with straps and bows.

I torture myself with shame for even thinking this in the privacy of my mind, but there are moments during these fits when I feel as though maybe life was easier before Ryland had sound. Before she could hear, Ryland was a typical toddler in regards to clothing: she let me dress her how I liked; she just didn't know any different because there were parts of her experience that she wasn't able to express just yet. Now, though, it's as though my daughter is a completely different child. With each passing day, Ryland's language develops, and that leads to an increase in her confidence and her sense of self. It seems that sound has given her more tools to understand the world and in turn, express herself. She's beginning to understand that she can have an opinion.

One day in early 2011 while we're shopping in Kohl's, I assume that she's a little confused when she gravitates toward the little boys' section. "I wan dis, Momma," she says, pointing to a three-piece suit. Her voice is little but assertive, and she looks up at me expectantly.

"Ry, no honey, you don't need that. Come on, let's go home!" My urgency isn't so much due to our rush to actually arrive at our house; it's that I know Ryland's sense of determination. Something about her attraction to this section makes me certain that it would be hard to tear her away.

As I think about it, it occurs to me that on Sunday mornings while I thumb through the newspaper advertisements to look for sales, Ryland often sits with me and circles what toys she would like. Recently, I've noticed that she pays no attention to the Hello Kitty and My Little Pony toys—instead, she's been asking about toys that to me seem to have been made for boys. After she's in bed, I've just thrown away the ad and not worried about having to actually buy the toy. But here, inside the department store, is the first time she's ever expressed her interest in boys' things in public. As she lingers, looking up at this suit on the rack, it worries me that we'll face an embarrassing temper tantrum.

"Come on," I repeat. "Let's go home and see Daddy."

To that, she finally agrees.

The experience stays with me for the days to follow. Nothing serious, I suppose, but still, it felt strange. A couple of weeks later, I'm searching for her in all the usual places Ryland's bedroom, the kitchen, even out in the front yard.

"Ryland!" I call out, beginning to panic. "Kobe, where's Ryland?" I run back inside the house. "Ry? Ryland!" And all the way at the end of the hall, in my bedroom, I find her:

She's hiding in the closet, wearing one of Jeff's shirts.

"Ryland?"

She turns to me, and on her face is a smile from ear to ear. Then she takes note of what must be an alarmed reaction on my face. "Momma," she says. "Please don't tell anybody."

Her shame crushes my heart, and I'm not sure who's more confused: Ryland, or me.

This humiliation coming from innocent Ryland is completely alarming to me—a huge red flag. *Please don't tell anyone about this.* Ryland is a smart kid. She's been picking up more and more on our comments and the social cues around her. She knows that she receives praise for certain things that adults consider "cute," but suddenly, she's starting to recognize that other things make us feel uncomfortable.

I make a point to pay even more attention over the next few weeks, and anytime she's gone from sight for more than a couple of minutes, I know just where to look. For a while, it's actually kind of precious to find her trying on Jeff's work boots, shirts, and ties. Is it that the materials of his clothes feel soft on her skin? Does she just like the scent of her daddy's shirts? Or maybe she likes things that button up in the front, since she has to take her cochlear implant devices off before we can slip anything over her head.

I don't see it as much other than a little girl developing "tomboy" tastes. *What's so wrong with that?* I think to myself. *You go, girl.*

But then her fascination evolves, and she begins to test us to see what we consider acceptable. When she asks for black-and-blue Vans sneakers at the outlet store and rips off her shirt to play in the pool, I begin to wonder if there's a little more to it than wanting to imitate the neighbor kids and the little boys she sees at her swim lessons.

And then, within a few weeks, every day as soon as we arrive home from school, she races back to Jeff's closet and plays dress-up for as long as I'll allow her. *It's not like we're out in public,* I reason with myself. *Maybe playing dress-up is a good way for her to develop her imagination.* I know that when I was a kid, I was much more interested in my mom's lipstick and high heels, but isn't that supposed to be one of the great lessons of parenthood—that your child isn't going to make all the same choices for themselves as you did throughout your life?

In a way, I'm really proud of Ryland for being so low-maintenance and sporty, but when some of Jeff's good collared shirts and trousers start to get dirty and frayed from Ry dragging herself around the house in them, I stand in the middle of his closet and think. *Okay. Now, this is getting to be a problem.*

Around this time, a former coworker from the dental office delivers a box of clothes that her granddaughter has outgrown. Ryland and I unpack the box of clothes in her bedroom, and among the bright-colored tops and dresses is a Burberry blouse—its famous tan, black, and red plaid magnetizing Ryland's attention. "Dis, Momma," Ryland points, as I'm folding the clothes into her dresser drawers.

"Do you want to try the skirt that goes with it?"

"No. Dis."

I unfold the shirt and put it on her. The next day, she asks to wear it again, and then again, and the request continues incessantly. As the weeks and then the months go on, she fights more, and more . . . and more . . . to wear outfits similar to this. In time, I see a pattern as clear as the Burberry print: it is only in the more masculine-styled clothes that Ryland will exit the house in peace.

Following this, on the days that I dare to put her in something else, I begin to draw an association between this and her ongoing habit of wetting herself; Ryland knows that if she has an accident in a particular outfit, then I'll take it off her, and will sometimes be forced to throw it away for good. I begin to tote not just pull-ups, baby wipes, and extra underwear in my diaper bag—an accessory that I'm not even sure is appropriate for the mother of a three-and-a-half-year-old to be hauling—but I also carry multiple outfits at a time (along, of course, with spare batteries for her ears).

The only way to solve it is to give in. I'm so overwhelmed with my task of trying to teach Ryland language that I don't have enough patience to figure out why she's refusing girls' clothes. I just try to keep Ryland happy, whatever that means at any given moment. When we're at home, she takes any opportunity she can to be shirtless. She takes a liking to plain T-shirts or shorts in solid colors of blue, beige, and white. *I have a tomboy for a daughter,* I say to myself with a shrug.

At moments, typically in the peace and privacy of our home, I'm thrilled that she feels so fierce in who she is and lives with such confidence, but I'd be lying to anyone if I said that managing her image—okay, *our* image—with others doesn't come with some conflict. I know it sounds selfish, but every parent wants his or her child to be complimented and noticed for being adorable. Unfortunately, compliments don't come as easily when your daughter looks like a boy with unmanaged, long, wild hair hanging down from under her Chargers ball cap. The compliments were endless when Ryland was a baby and small toddler—her dress matched her shoes and her bow. But those days are long over, and by the looks of things, I'm not sure I'll ever be that mom with the prettily dressed little girl.

Deep down, we all care a little what others think of us. I think it's natural to want to be seen in a positive light, whatever that might mean, and this goes for the way others see our children, as well. I'll be the first to admit: I do it, too. Whenever I see a little kid with long, dirty fingernails or dirty ears, I can't help but think to myself, *Does his or her parent not care about keeping their kid clean and groomed?*

Fearing this kind of judgment from other adults, a growing part of me avoids leaving the house with Ryland. On days when Jeff is working, it's impossible for me to talk her out of her insistence, and I've been caving in to let her wear boy clothes around town while I pick up a few groceries or run to the post office. I want Ryland to be happy, and I can tell being seen in public in her "dress-up clothes" makes her feel this way.

I ask myself: Whom *exactly* do I care to impress? The grocery clerk? The dry cleaning receptionist? Why is it okay for Ryland to express herself at home, but then be forced to change when we leave the house? What am I not teaching her about being herself in the face of others' opinions?

Knowing that he's aware of this to some degree but processing the whole thing in his own quiet way, I hesitate to lean on Jeff about it too heavily, but it's in situations this significant that I need him most, and that he's always so logical and wise. However, I also know that we both witness Ryland's happiness when we allow her to wear the clothes that she chooses. One night, I broach the question with him carefully.

"Jeff . . . what do you think about all of this?"

"Think about what?" he replies.

Great start. "About Ryland, and how she is at home. I know that you don't see it all the time, but the second she gets home, she runs off and changes into boy stuff."

"I know," he says. "I see it, and as far as I'm concerned, I don't mind what she does when she's at home."

Whew, I think to myself. At least we're on the same page with that—if I had to start enforcing anything different, I wouldn't even want to be at home. "With the implants," he says, "she already has so much to deal with, and she has to work so hard. If coming home and dressing like that makes her happy, then I'm okay with it." There's a brief pause . . . then he continues. "But . . . I still think we need to implement some discipline about her clothes when she's out of the house. With the attention she already gets from the implants, I'm not sure I'm ready to answer questions about why she's always dressed like a boy around town."

"Okay," I tell him. We agree: we'll just let Ryland be whoever she wants at home.

We use this judiciousness when it comes to what she wears out, sometimes bribing her with toys and candy if she puts up a fight against a girly outfit. (I know it's not A-plus parenting, but I also know every parent has done it on one occasion or another.) On Thanksgiving, Christmas, and then Easter, we still insist that she wears clothes that were made for girls. But for casual, everyday outings and school, as she turns up more and more in long-sleeved T-shirts and her trademark Vans, most everybody who knows her praises her for being herself. "She's cool!" Jeff's brothers say, and Jeff and I smile and go along. "She's comfy," I tell them, or, "At least she matches." Some members of our family look on and turn their heads, saying very little. With a glance and a grimace toward Ryland out of the corner of her eye, my cousin Melissa says, "Yikes. Maybe she'll outgrow it." I feel pain inside that they can't see the positive side of this—that I'm a mom who will do anything to see my child happy, or that I'm trying to strike a compromise with Ryland by continuing to style her hair with ponytails, braids, and bows.

It's impossible for me to get my head around how anyone who loves Ryland would allow their judgment to cloud their opinions of us and our efforts to do what's right for our child and keep peace in our household. I've been convinced that following my instincts as a mom is the right thing to do, but around certain members of our family, I find myself shrinking back inside: should I be *trying* to get Ryland to conform? On one occasion, Peg and Rand ask if they can take Ryland on a mini-vacation for a couple of days. When Jeff and I agree, they also ask if they can come over and pack Ryland's bag for the trip. My heart drops. I'm surprised by this request, and it's painfully obvious that they have concerns over Ryland's clothing and appearance.

Of course it's Jeff who gets the brunt of my hurt and frustration. As the scenario swells, it drives a wedge between my husband and me, and I find myself looking forward to the nights when Jeff works and Ryland and I are home alone, free to hang out and not worry about pleasing anyone else.

These family members just don't know the daily standoffs that go on inside our home and how painful this problem is becoming for all of us. Only silently, after these relatives are out of sight, do I allow their reactions to collapse my emotions.

I start to catch Ryland looking at clothing catalogs and admiring the boys who are dressed in three-piece suits. She stares at them, mesmerized by how handsome they are in their dapper little outfits. "I don't know where she gets this," I tell Jeff.

"I know," he agrees. Jeff is handsome and well dressed, but he readily admits that he rarely has reason to put on a suit. "She only ever sees me in my fire uniform," he says. We continue to wonder why our daughter is drawn to the most masculine outfits imaginable.

I CONTINUE TO shop for clothes in the girls' department, but I spend hours there looking for the plainest cuts and colors. Ryland will locate the tag of any piece of apparel I hold up and search it for any hint of pink or a girly logo. If she finds it, she simply states, "I don't like that." She pushes away all pink and purple, any dress or skirt, and even pajamas that look feminine.

During one Target outing with Ryland, it's her joy that finally tips the scale to bring about the first instance when I ever actually buy my daughter clothes that were made for a boy. As I push our cart past the boys' section, Ryland's eyes light up: she's spotted a blue, long-sleeved shirt with a collar. Seeing that it's on the clearance rack, I approach it and lift the tag. *Seven dollars.* I weigh the happiness of my child against a silly seven dollars. *What could it hurt?* In fact, Jeff might actually thank me for *saving* money, since Ryland has continued to damage his clothes.

When we arrive at home, she runs immediately into her bedroom and puts it on, buttons perfectly straight, no help necessary. Instantly it's Ryland's favorite piece of clothing. I don't think I've ever seen her this happy.

Wanting Ryland to grow up like every other Southern California kid, in the midst of our tomboy saga Jeff and I enroll her in swim lessons with Gianna. We go together to the first one, collaborating carefully to take off her external hearing devices and put plugs in her ears to protect her tubes, followed by a swim cap to keep everything in place. The instructor is completely cooperative about the fact that Ryland can't communicate while swimming other than with sign language, and for half an hour we watch her from lounge chairs and we converse with other parents, who have questions about Ryland's need for ASL.

Ryland takes beautifully to the water; it's as though it's a quiet sanctuary for her—a secure place of peace.

I begin to take her to the lessons on my own. Most of the time, Jenn is beside me during class, and I always update her on my latest saga, which usually has to do with Ryland fighting me out of girls' clothing—*especially* swimsuits. One day, I'm seated next to a swim mom whom I know only relatively well.

"It's not that Ryland doesn't want to swim," I tell her. "I mean look at her—she loves the water. I don't know," I say with a sigh. "She fights me anytime I try to put something girly on her. I think she may be a lesbian one day."

Only after I've heard the words do I realize that I've mused this out loud. The other mom looks at me as if I've just sprouted a second head, then turns her gaze to the pool, where she keeps her eyes fixed for the rest of the lesson. I can feel her judgment of me, her assumption that some kind of force could get Ryland to bend and fit what the adults around her want. I can almost hear her saying, "Get some control of your kid and put on the darn dress!" *My gosh,* I try to tell myself, *it was just a comment—how could I really know what Ryland's sexual preference will be?* I was sharing my parental instinct with this woman, but also, maybe without knowing it, I was testing her response. I was looking for someone, *anyone,* to confirm what's going on with my child. One thing I know for sure: no matter what, I'll always love Ryland.

At this point, unaware of what else could be happening, I automatically link Ryland's gender expression with what her future sexual preference might be—my early assumptions with Ryland's masculine presentation have simply been that she may grow up to be attracted to women. I've always believed that sexuality is determined by genetics, at least in part, so I always had an idea in the back of my head that we could have a gay child because we have that in our family. Granted, I know Ryland isn't having any strong attractions at this age, but it's definitely something I've considered. It seems a bit strange to think of a three-year-old's sexual choices, but seeking out a label for her at this age somehow makes me feel just a little more secure about what's been going on.

At this point, it's very clear that I can't confide about my questions and experiences with just anyone, and I find Jeff and myself growing a little more selective about the people we spend time with—increasingly, only people who are both loving and well-informed tend to be the most compassionate and welcoming of our daughter. If we make plans to spend extended amounts of time with anyone, it's generally our families—and more than ever, I find myself turning to my parents for their strength and parenting wisdom. Sometimes, in the middle of the night, I tiptoe out to the computer and let the tears roll down my face as I write novel-length emails to my mom in search of what she would do in the different incidents I'm facing. First thing the next morning, she always answers, telling me that she believes there is a greater plan for Ryland and that if I pray, God will hear me and strengthen me.

My parents recommend that I make time to go back to church to be part of a community and pray for some answers, but a church is really the last place I want to go with questions about my child's sexual orientation. I'm afraid there will be too much judgment there, and I don't want to be swayed into any particular way of thinking. In our family, love is unconditional and universal.

One of Jenn's friends hears about Ryland's love for male

clothes and sends us a box of her son's hand-me-downs. Ryland and I peek inside, and Ry looks up at me with those big, hazel eyes: the box is stuffed with Gap shirts, sweatshirts, pairs of long pants. These definitely aren't like much of the rest of Ryland's wardrobe—girls' clothes neutralized in shades of blue, green, and yellow. These are definitely clothes for a boy, and as her options grow, so does her insistence. Ryland fights to wear these boys' clothes everywhere.

At preschool, Ryland's teacher introduces her class to a math and phonics website called Starfall.com, where the kids can design their own avatar's face and clothing and play from anywhere. We log in at home, and together Ryland and I begin to make choices for her character. The program asks us: is our avatar a boy or a girl? "Girl," I click.

"I am a *BOY!*" Ryland screams.

I look at my child, deep in the eyes. I don't think I can fight this anymore. I need help.

Why am I even fighting her? When I force myself to really think about it, I realize that I've been denying the truth about her true well-being *again*. I had been in denial once before with Ryland's deafness. It cost us months of setback and potential limits for Ryland's hearing success, and once we got through the worst of it, I promised myself that I would never make that mistake again. I'm paying attention to the signs this time . . . it's just that I don't know what the signs and all of her struggle mean.

Slowly, I'm discovering that there's something even deeper to this expression of masculinity. I start to listen to Ryland from around the corner while she's playing Starfall. Sometimes, when I walk into the room, she turns to me quickly and her face flushes with embarrassment. One day, when I find her playing, she looks at me with those same innocent eyes as on the day when I found her in Jeff's closet and she asked me, *"Momma, please don't tell anybody."* I realize: I cannot fuel Ryland's feelings of shame, or make her feel a sense of responsibility for how I as her mother feel. I know that this won't be easy, but if this is really who my child is, then I need to learn how not just to tolerate it, but to *embrace* that.

Chapter Five

Immediate Attention

During this period, Ryland is going on four years old and now transitioning out of the special needs preschool because her speech and language have progressed so quickly. Our fears associated with her deafness are starting to ease, and we are extremely active throwing large gatherings for the Bionic Ear Association. We also have new families of deaf children over for dinner to be a source of support for them, but even in the presence of the families who relate to our journey with Ryland's hearing and speaking, there is a constant, pulsing anxiety inside me over Ryland's masculine behaviors and expression. I don't know where all this is headed, and as a first-time mom, I definitely don't know how to manage it with any sort of expertise.

As much as I can, I soak in every possible moment to observe Ryland being carefree and happy. I love to stand back and watch her fondness for different things develop: she adores animals, exploring outside, being silly, using her hands, being creative, and playing with her friends. Gianna is the pal she sees the most frequently—they always get along, and their personalities complement each other. Both are take-charge, but when it comes down to it, Gianna tends to let Ryland take the lead. When Jenn and I take them swimming, Gianna wears a ruffled pink swimsuit while Ryland, still wearing a ponytail, refuses to wear anything besides blue swimming bottoms. She and Gianna carry on with no worries, loving all the make-believe scenarios and games. Jeff, Jenn, and I marvel in amazement when, while they're playing House, Gianna completely goes with the flow when Ryland tells her: "I be da dad."

"Okay!"

They race back to Ryland's room to pick out dress-up clothes. Gianna finds the frilliest pink tutu, and Ryland grabs her blue shirt. (She'd also begun to request the addition of a necktie, so I bought a few kids' ties with elastic bands to go over her head, which she's been pairing with a T-shirt at home.)

In August 2011, Ryland starts at a local preschool. It's a well-known, highly regarded program in our neighborhood that's connected to Foothills, the Methodist church in our area. The preschool there is known for its safety and warm environment. All of our neighbors' kids attend, and Jeff and I feel that it would be nice for Ryland, and also for us, to be part of a school community with so many local friends.

Last year, the special needs school was a supportive environment for Ryland—they coached her on the name of her teachers and classmates to make sure she knew what to call them, to avoid getting lost in the shuffle. They always double-checked to be sure she heard her instructions clearly. They even carpeted the classroom so that the children with cochlear implants could pick up the best acoustical sound possible. But now, at Foothills, we're excited for Ryland to be challenged in an environment with typically developing children, too. I don't say this to anyone but Jeff, but Ryland's participation at Foothills makes it feel as though we've arrived. Finally, we're a normal family.

At our orientation meeting, I make a point to let Ryland's new teacher know that not only is Ryland deaf with cochlear implants, but she's also a tomboy who may very well hang around the boys more than the girls. The word *tomboy* is the quickest, easiest way I can find to describe Ryland and protect her from people's expectations that she will like "girl" things, and I find myself beginning to use it as much for my protection from judgment as for Ryland's. It upsets my child so much every time a teacher or nurse or anyone else assumes she will want the princess sticker over the car sticker. When teachers hand out projects, or ask children to line up in the girl line or the boy line, they sometimes don't think about how uncomfortable this may be for kids like Ryland, who are more gender-fluid. At Ryland's special needs preschool, many times I watched as she struggled to find a way to politely choose something that wasn't offered to her as a choice, or to turn down a toy or an opportunity altogether because it just didn't suit her. Now, as she enters her mainstream preschool, I can't help but feel like I have to step in and help her in these cases. Why is it that we, as a society, automatically assume what a girl or boy likes before they even get the opportunity to figure it out for themselves and choose?

Ms. Vicci is a woman in her fifties, young-looking with brown hair and a kind smile. "We'll all watch her closely," she assures us, "and we'll roll with it. Every child is different."

We are over the moon when we attend our first parent-teacher conference and learn that Ryland is able to communicate and understand at a level with other children her same age. It's a miracle, really, and it makes me feel like all the pain we've been through is worth it.

As the school year continues, I grow friendly with some of the mothers who have children in Ryland's class. I take a liking to Chase's mom—a sweet single mom with a heart of gold in whom I've confided some of my questions about Ryland's sexuality. Chase is also one of the nicest little boys I've ever met. He's a beautiful child—very tall with olive skin, a precious smile, and the most gorgeous brown curls. He also has mild autism. His mom often sends him to school with small treats that they baked together at home for him to share with Ryland. Because Chase grows so fast for his age, they give Ryland boxes of his hand-me-down clothes. One day he even brings Ryland a school folder that matches his own with the infamous red Angry Bird on the cover.

Chase and his mom share a home with Chase's grandmother, Barbara, who is Chase's daytime caregiver. At school pickup, I often chat with Barbara, loving her spirit—she's an activist, she tells me, and I've noticed that she has a bumper sticker on her car that reads "99%." I was raised conservative, but I know how to listen and I enjoy hearing her outspoken views on politics and social issues. I respect her and her passion, and I'm intrigued by her dedication to her beliefs. Most of all, I see how much she loves her grandson, and I don't really care what political party she chooses.

One day after school, Ryland and I are at their house. Barbara and I are in the kitchen talking when Ryland runs out and puts her hands on my lap. "Momma," she says, "I go potty."

"You have to go potty?" I ask her, glancing down. "Oh, you already *did* go potty. Uh-oh."

Immediately, Chase's grandma waltzes back to Chase's room and brings out a pair of Chase's Star Wars underwear.

Ryland's eyes light up like the Fourth of July.

We go to the bathroom and change into them. The underwear has a blue background and a red waistband, with black Darth Vader faces and the Star Wars logo. On our way out, I hug Barbara.

"Thanks for the underwear," I tell her. "We'll return them."

"Please," she says, "don't worry about it. We can spare a pair of underwear for Ryland."

When Jeff comes home, I tell him the story about Ryland's potty accident and the Darth Vader underwear. He takes it in, folds his arms, and stands back against the kitchen counter. In his reaction, I see a disappointment—no, a sadness—that I haven't seen until now. He looks at me, and with our silence, we acknowledge it.

"This may be one step too far," he says.

"You think I'm encouraging this?"

"You're allowing it."

"Allowing what?"

"You're allowing her to be in charge!"

"What do you want me to do instead?"

"Something!" he says. "Now it will be even harder to—"

"To what, Jeff?" I know what he's saying: now it will be even harder to curb some of this behavior.

I know my husband does not like the idea of his daughter wearing boys' undies, and I know that I should be able to stop it. Parents should have control over their children's wardrobes, right? But nobody, not even Jeff, knows the fight I go through every day. I've tried *everything*, and besides giving in, nothing I've been able to think of has worked.

I can see where Jeff is coming from, but I don't know what to do about it. We may have just reached the point of no return.

The next day, I wash the Star Wars underwear, still intending to return them to Chase, but Ryland asks to wear them again. I bargain with myself: because they were borrowed, we can get away with letting Ryland wear them, can't we? We put them on, and Ryland wants to wear them again, the next day. I wash them again and again, over and over. Ryland refuses to wear anything else. I wash them until they fade to baby blue and I can barely make out the Darth Vader faces. Does it bother me that my daughter likes boys' underwear? Some. But her daily wardrobe tantrums bother me worse. Her not being able to hear bothers me worse than that.

To everyone else, I'm supposed to have this child under control, but Ryland is very strong, self-aware, and clear on what she wants. Plus, in my eyes, she's not being *disobedient*—she's generally an incredibly sweet and loving child who's considerate of others, and she listens in every other situation except where her clothes are concerned. She just expresses who she is through her external appearance, like all of us. *She wants to dress like a boy.*

I know that for Jeff, especially working in such a macho field of work, this is growing more and more uncomfortable all the time. I also believe that if the rest of the family were to find out how far this has gone behind closed doors, they would find it very strange and awkward. Our little Ryland in boys' underwear? I get how something about it is just too close for comfort.

A FEW MONTHS later, we learn that we're expecting again. Jeff and I are thrilled, and so is Ryland—she's been asking for a sibling for months. However, because of all I went through in my first pregnancy, I hold some trepidation that I don't hide very well. My doctor tells me to put my feet up and relax as much as I can, and it's all I can do not to laugh in his face: I have a three-and-a-half-year-old to keep up with, a house to take care of, a husband who comes home exhausted after twenty-four-hour shifts, and extended family who need us, too. Relaxing won't really be an option.

Periodically throughout the first trimester, Melissa comes to help take care of me, putting her nursing skills to the test as I fight to hold any morsel of food in my stomach without losing it moments later. I hit midterm, twenty weeks, just as we're nearing Ryland's fourth birthday. Jeff and I have discussed it: we don't want to throw her a birthday party this year because we don't know how we'll manage her disappointment over receiving "girl" gifts. I don't want to have to explain to every single guest that Ryland is a tomboy, and I feel very awkward addressing what presents people should buy for her. She would be so sad to open presents that are designed in the traditional way for little girls. We feel like we're protecting her by making sure she won't have to deal with that, but we're aware that we're also actively thinking of depriving Ryland of a birthday party because of our own insecurities and uncertainties.

It's a tough call . . . until I have a brainstorm: my parents used to love to take my brother and me to Disneyland every year before Christmas, and Ryland is at the perfect age to bring back that tradition. Jeff agrees with me that this could be a good way to avoid an uncomfortable situation, and the outcome is what matters to us the most. If we can get Ryland on board for a Disneyland birthday, then the deferment of a party could help keep the peace for everyone.

"Ry," I ask her, "for your birthday, how would you like it if we go to Disneyland? Grandma and Grandpa will come along, and you can choose a friend to bring with you—what do you think?"

She tilts her head in consideration, and then shouts, "Yeah!" She chooses to bring Gianna, and we all gear up to celebrate Ryland's big day at the happiest place on earth. I choose a sundress, knowing that Gianna will be dressed to the Disneyland nines, and knowing that when we arrive, every Disney princess at every intersection of the park will greet Ryland. I don't want our whole family to stand witness to what happens when her outfit creates confusion.

As we're getting ready for my parents and Gianna to arrive, Ryland fights me on the outfit choice. Hard. Jeff tries to reason with her while I stand back, and when he looks at me with surrender on his face, I attempt to negotiate with candy, then toys. When neither of those options works, I remember: I am the parent!

Our reasoning turns into a wrestle as I try to wrangle her into the dress. Ryland is sobbing, tears and saliva smeared all over her face. "I don't want to go!" she wails. "I don't want to go, *I don't like this!*"

Suddenly, I feel a hardening sensation in my tummy and I recognize the contractions instantly: these are preterm labor pains. *I should go sit on the couch,* I tell myself, but I should also do Ryland's hair, stick in a bow, and brush her teeth before my parents get here.

Never imagining that a child would dare miss Disneyland be-cause of a dress (and not wanting to disappoint my parents, who have been planning this day for weeks), I compromise with Ry: if she'll wear a gray T-shirt and jeans—*with* hair bows—then we can still go. She calms down and agrees. Heading into the bath room to finish getting her ready, I stop myself in our hallway to make sure: the contractions have stopped, but I am worried sick. *Going to Disneyland is probably the last thing I should be doing today,* I think. I promise myself that I'll take rests throughout the day and definitely the second that I feel something more.

When we make it to the park, Ryland has pretty much forgot-ten the whole sundress episode. Before we enter the turnstiles into the park, we head straight to Goofy's Kitchen for a special breakfast buffet to celebrate Ry's big day. Then as we make our way into the park, she is visibly standoffish when Cinderella and Ariel say things like, "What a pretty girl you are!" Instead, she's got her heart set on the Darth Vader training academy. It's this cute little Disneyland skit where the Jedi Knights select kids out of the crowd to go through training to eventually engage in a swordfight with Darth Vader.

I know how badly Ryland wants to be chosen; she's been talk-ing about it for weeks. She and Gianna stand among the audi-ence of kids, the two of them jumping and waving to be chosen. Gianna couldn't care less about Star Wars, but when she looks around at Ryland and all the other kids' excitement, she jumps and waves even more to keep up.

As the Jedi Knights make their selections, I notice that they're choosing children significantly older than Ryland and Gianna, most likely so they're old enough to follow commands. Suddenly, a Jedi chooses Gianna. I freeze. *Oh God, please choose Ryland, please choose Ryland!* It's her birthday, and it will kill Ryland if Gianna gets chosen and she doesn't! I grab Ryland's hand and lift her up so that the Jedi can see her, and finally, one of the kind Jedis motions for Ryland to come onstage. Ryland runs for the stage, and her eyes light up as she performs in front of the crowd. She and Gianna are the tiniest ones performing by far, but Ryland's smile is bigger than anything onstage.

Ry and Gianna are still buzzing about this when, nearing lunchtime, I see a man who seems to be approaching us. He's wearing a button-down shirt, a hat, and sunglasses, and at his side is a blond woman who's walking toward us, too.

"Tim?" he says, removing his sunglasses.

My dad stops in his tracks. "Eric?"

"Pastor Eric!"

There are hugs all around with our old family friend and his wife, Karen, neither of whom we've seen since he was gracious enough to travel with our family to Oregon to conduct my brother's funeral service and help us spread Ryan's ashes near the lighthouse that stands near my grandfather's property, which has been one of our family's favorite places to visit over the years.

"Did you two just take the day off to come wander around Disneyland?" my dad teases.

"We did." Pastor Eric says, "Since our church is in Irvine, we decided to get Disney passes so we could come and wander Disneyland on our days off."

We all laugh. Pastor Eric and his wife join us for lunch while Ryland poses for my camera with a smile full of french fries, holding her birthday souvenir:

This certificate announces that
RYLAND
Has proven to be worthy of training to become a Jedi,
the guardians of peace and justice in the galaxy
From this day forth, remember, a Jedi uses the force
for knowledge and defense, never for attack.
The force will be with you, always.

The certificate is stamped by the Jedi Training Academy, and Disneyland.

When I check the photo in my digital display, it shows Pastor Eric and Karen giggling at Ryland in the background. "Little warrior in the making," Pastor Eric laughs.

I'm halfway tempted to tell him: *You have no idea.*

AFTER THE VISIT to Disneyland, my doctor orders immediate bed rest, where, he says, it's likely that I'll spend the entire remainder of the pregnancy. My anxiety spikes higher than ever, knowing that I'll need to depend more on our family to help with Ryland, which means that I'm going to lose control. But I know that if I don't take the doctor's instructions seriously, my second child's life could be gone.

The weeks to come grow in difficulty until they're finally filled with terror. Peg comes over throughout the week to pick up Ryland while I rest or shop for the family's Christmas gifts online. Peg cooperates patiently with Ryland when, at first, the male-oriented requests are pretty trivial: Ryland will only eat off blue-colored plates and drink out of blue cups. But she also begins to observe how Ryland absolutely will not wear a shirt in the house, and she takes note of the very masculine tendencies— playing with boys' toys (Shrek drives dinosaurs around in a red pickup truck in our house), making sound effects like a boy while she's playing . . . and even beginning to try to stand to go potty. Jeff and I have discussed the fact that the bathroom perpetually smells like it needs cleaning, until one day when I walk into the bathroom and find Ryland facing the toilet.

Again, that deer-in-the-headlights look of shame, but I'm not mad; instead, my heart sinks, and I'm just glad to finally have an answer to why the bathroom has smelled like urine.

"Honey?" I ask her gently. "What are you doing?"

"Nuffing," she says. She hoists up her pants and turns swiftly to the sink to wash her hands.

I watch her whiz past me to exit the bathroom and wonder if it's worthwhile just to let the incident go, feeling just as embarrassed as Ryland looked. I remember giggling as a little girl when my older brother told me that he stands up to pee, and, curious, I even tried it once or twice to see what it was like. I use this memory to try to brush off Ryland's potty incident as best I can, chalking it up to normal toddler experimentation, but within the next few weeks, I pay attention to how often I have to clean the area around the toilet. It's obvious that Ryland is using the toilet little-boy-style more than on the occasional test trial.

When my contractions randomly start again, Peg and Rand take Ryland to stay at their house for a couple of nights.

I pack a bag full of girl clothes, including some that Peg and Rand have given as gifts, in hopes that Ryland will cooperate with her grandparents more than she does with me, or, at the very least, that Peg will see that I really do make an attempt to dress Ryland in little girls' clothes.

When the contractions cease, and after I've gotten a couple of good days of rest, Peg brings Ryland back home.

"Hillary," she says, "I saw something that I can't seem to get out of my mind."

Dreading more, I ask her: "What's that?"

"When Ryland arrived at our house, she was wearing little boys' underwear."

Oh no. Ryland had dressed herself and put on the Star Wars underwear.

I start to defend myself, finagling an explanation, but Peg stares at me blankly—she's not at all amused. Struggling in vain to convince her that this is nothing, I resort to: "It's not like you can see them. I mean, they're under her clothes."

Silence. Awkwardness. No response.

She leaves quietly, and I am sick to my stomach. I guess I've pushed the limit. But someone had to stand up for Ryland, and it had to be me. I feel like they're blaming me for pushing Ryland toward a masculine identity, but this is *real*. This is all her. I know her better than anyone does. I never put her in day care and I have been extremely cautious about whom I've allowed to care for her. I'm with my child all the time. She was deaf, and I already feel that she needs me more than most children need their parents. I'm here to protect her . . . even if that means protecting her from the opinions of our own family. I know very well now where they all stand on boys' underwear.

Ryland is in bed when Jeff arrives home from work. He comes into the bedroom.

"You heard?"

"Yeah." Instead of looking at me, he clasps his hands behind his head and looks up at the ceiling, searching for an answer. "I heard."

"So they're upset?"

He heads into his closet and starts to undress. For a moment he's silent . . . and then over his shoulder, he tells me: "They didn't like it one bit."

PREGNANT, ANGRY, FRUSTRATED, and tired of disappointing everyone—especially Jeff and Ryland—as Christmas nears, I give up and put Jeff in charge of picking out Ryland's Christmas outfit.

"I'll let you take over," I tell him. "I'm always stuck between trying to make her happy and trying to make you and everyone else happy, and I'm exhausted of taking the heat for her. You'll see what I'm dealing with every day." We argue constantly over Ryland's appearance and the concerns of those with whom we are constantly surrounded. I feel like everyone critiques what I'm doing wrong, but nobody helps or offers any chance of a solution. I feel resentful, like he should be taking on this challenge with me, instead of letting me face the wolves all alone.

Initially, Jeff thinks he can handle Ryland's Christmas clothing situation easily. "No problem," he says, and it's all I can do not to say, *Just you wait.* He's the man of the house, the enforcer, the boss—the voice that Ryland listens to the most. I know he believes that I let Ryland get away with way too much of this dressing nonsense. Now he'll see for himself.

Jeff spends an evening searching the Internet, looking for an outfit we can agree on. Eventually we come across an image of Brad Pitt and Angelina Jolie's family and take note that one of their children is a gender-nonconforming natal female like Ryland. *Finally!* We've found a child with a "style" that can work for Ryland: a white, long-sleeved, button-up shirt, short black vest, a tie, and black jeans. When Jeff sees this look, something finally clicks for him. "Some girls rock the vest look," he says cheerfully, and we agree that this is a perfect compromise.

It's so refreshing for us to see a child in the public eye who wears the tomboy look like we hope Ryland can! We want her to feel good about herself and her clothes, but also to fit in with societal expectations. We're learning that unfortunately, you can't always have both . . . but to see images of John Jolie-Pitt (who was called Shiloh at the time) for us, is a good start. For the first time ever on this topic, we're all on the same page. It's actually exciting to have an idea that we've all agreed on.

Feeling a renewed confidence, Jeff takes Ryland shopping for an outfit that includes a collared shirt and a vest, like Brad and Angelina's child. From the sofa, I watch them as they head out the front door in hopes that this will be a fun day of shopping and bonding.

When they reach the store, Jeff texts me: he realizes it isn't as easy to find these pieces as he thought it would be, especially that Ryland agrees on. Finally, he's subject to what I've been dealing with, and when Ryland leads him to the boys' department, the two of them manage to piece together an outfit that Ryland is more than happy to wear. From the dressing room, Jeff texts pictures to me. Ry looks super-cute in vests and Ralph Lauren Polo shirts—and, I notice, appears so happy in the photos!

After they leave the store, Jeff takes Ryland to speech therapy in Poway. It's a long trip and an intense hour of therapy, so a four-year-old looks forward to a Happy Meal– or smoothie-worthy ride home. While they listen to music, Ryland throws one of her hair bows up front—something that she knows would not be okay with me. The bows are the one final piece of wardrobe compromise that I've negotiated.

"Ry," Jeff says. "Why did you do that?"

"I don't want to wear them anymore."

Treading lightly and now very curious, Jeff takes the conversation where it seems to be heading next.

"Ryland," he says, "do you just like playing with boy toys, or are you a girl who wants to be a boy?"

Ryland hesitates. She's aware of what her answer should be, and she doesn't want to raise any more questions from Dad. "A girl who likes boy things," she responds.

"Okay," Jeff says, satisfied with Ryland's answer. Still, he senses that there is a deeper truth that he as the father should dig for. "Would you want to cut your hair and look like Daddy?"

Ryland nods her head in excitement. *Yes!*

"So, you want short hair—you want to cut your long hair?"

"Yeah!"

I'm still resting on the couch when they arrive at home. Jeff is somewhere else . . . distracted. I can tell he's upset.

"What's wrong, honey?"

"Oh," he says, shaking his head. "Not much."

"No, really," I ask him. "What's wrong?"

"Tell you in a little while," he whispers. "After we put Ry to bed."

After Ryland is asleep, we go into our office, which functions as a spare bedroom with a double bed set up for guests. We lie down together, and Jeff's eyes fill with tears. I never see him cry. I never see him this upset. "What's wrong, babe?"

"Ryland . . ." he says. "Ryland told me she wants to cut her hair and be like me. I am scared. I am really scared. Something is different, Hill—something is going on!"

"I know, I know." I cradle his head into my chest. He cries like a baby as I hold him to me tightly. I've been walking a fine line with him because he has not been ready to accept this, but now it's all hit him. I have longed to have the big conversation with him about Ryland. I've used what we learned from denying her deafness not to make the same mistake here in a way that could permanently damage our little girl's self-perception, and I've been listening to what she's been expressing to strengthen my capacity to love my child for who she is. I saw my brother suffer his whole life trying to figure out how in the world to love himself. . . . I don't want that same life for my child.

Out of fear for Jeff's reactions and his personal denial around this subject, I've done everything I can to avoid it completely. Every time it's come up, I've felt his tension and have been waiting for him to bring it up first. Now, finally, the moment is here. Ryland has finally confessed to him what she's been feeling.

I'm proud of her, and also of Jeff for not shying away from the talk . . . but I'm also very, very scared for our child. What does this all mean?

We're afraid, confused. I've suspected Ryland would most likely be a member of the LGBTQ community, but I've simply imagined her as a lesbian. Both Jeff and I would accept and love her that way, or any way. Jeff's brother Scott has expanded our whole family's tolerance. Jeff's aunt Sue is also gay, and Rand

and Peg have kept her looped in on all that's been going on with Ryland. If there's any family, and any extended family, that could embrace a homosexual child, it's ours. But is there something else? Something inside tells me that we may be dealing with something more.

Chapter Six

Growing Family

I feel overwhelmed—crazy, even—to be thinking of Ryland's sexuality at age four, but Jeff and I are both very confused. I try to envision how long it's reasonable for a little girl to pass as a tomboy, until spring 2012, when Ryland draws a pre-school picture of herself as a little boy. It's further evidence that Ryland perceives herself to be male, and while the self-portrait is adorable, we don't really know how to explain it to anyone else. There's something else going on inside Ryland, and I have to dig deeper than sexual orientation. Ryland is so little. This is different than an attraction to the same sex this is Ryland telling us that she is incongruent with her physical body.

In early March 2012, my doctor finds that I've begun to dilate and forbids me to do anything except rest for what we antici-pate will be the final month of my pregnancy. I feel helpless and very emotional as I watch Jeff, his parents, and his brothers share care of Ryland. At this point, there's almost nothing I can do for my child . . . my child who needs me right now. Ryland seems like she is doing fine—her uncle Jay does a great job keeping her busy at the Birch Aquarium, the arcade for games and pizza and at surf lessons at the beach—but there are so many tasks that come with watching her that I fear she isn't getting everything she needs when she's out of my care. There are a lot of nuts and bolts that need attending to: her cochlear implants need to be cleaned and the batteries charged nightly, and in the morning there is a fifteen-minute routine to connect her ears to the FM transmitter for school. It's a long, tedious task on top of everything else, and I know it's a lot to ask of Jeff's family. It makes me uneasy to know the maintenance that's necessary with Ryland.

Her Nana and Papa are spoiling her, and so are her amazing uncles, and I know she has fun with all of them . . . but before they whisk her off, she hugs me for long periods. She isn't angry with me for not being able to be there, since she understands there is a baby inside me, and her apparent understanding of this only amplifies the guilt I feel for not doing my job as I'm usually able to do.

Doing all he can to keep me sane, Jeff manages to keep up with the laundry, dishes, grocery shopping, and bills. He also rearranges the living room for me to finish out my bed rest in as pleasing an atmosphere as possible. Ryland stands by as Jeff remounts the television to go above the fireplace and moves the couch and all the family pictures that hang on our walls. When he's finished, the room's been set up so that I can look out the window for these last few weeks until the second baby arrives. Jeff and Ryland—dressed in her John Jolie-Pitt–inspired vest— surround me (and my belly) when Peg snaps a photo of the three of us on my birthday, sitting inside their renovation and preparing to blow out the candles on my cake. We're all smiling hugely: me, feeling very loved and pleased, while the two of them appear so proud of their work.

It's in this final period of my pregnancy—when I'm forced to sit still instead of do *anything* to run the house—that I begin to search for resources that can enlighten me about Ryland's situation. I order books by gender experts and psychotherapists who specialize in child development, and there are prevailing themes that begin to encourage me to think completely differently about our situation.

One is that gender identity and sexuality are not one and the same. Ryland's inclination to live her life as a boy actually is completely apart from which gender—or genders—she may gravitate toward romantically. At first, this makes me scratch my head: could this *get* any more confusing? But it occurs to me that Ryland's sexual preference isn't something that we need to address or even fully understand for at least a few years. For now, this is a huge relief.

Another answer I find is that indeed we are just toddlers when we know who we are from a gender standpoint—that is, we're gender identified between ages two and five. *So that's why the clothing struggles started right after the cochlear implants,* I realize. It was the increased self-awareness that gaining sound gave her, *along with* the fact that we just so happened to have the procedure done at the same point in her life that a child's gender identification begins to form. According to what I'm reading, much of how a child expresses who he or she is is played out through their clothing choices. This is the period in our lives when we determine the way we'll want to dress, how we'll carry ourselves, and the person we'll grow into as we grow older and then into adulthood. So much of a person's long-term development takes place in this phase—cognitive, linguistic, physical, social, emotional, and more. It's very possible that the Ryland of today is who Ryland will be for life.

To be a tomboy is just a phase, and what we've been dealing with is definitely more than a phase. Phases end, and this tomboy thing is not ending—instead, over time, it's growing much stronger. My child's masculinity is deeply embedded in who Ryland is. I read that the difference between a transgender kid and a tomboy is that tomboys are okay with their physical body—they like being girls who do boyish things. Ryland's not like that. Instead, she is showing us more and more that she would prefer to have the body of a boy. She also follows the three criteria that I'm learning about in these books: she's insistent, consistent, and persistent, and she's been this way for more than three years. This masculine presentation has lingered very persistently, and it shows no signs of going away anytime soon. As I read, it dawns on me that there may be something much more to Ryland's self-perception. Maybe Ryland is right—maybe on the inside, in her brain and in her heart, she really is a boy.

Another point I read that brings me more clarity is stark: a statistic I find states that 41 percent of people who are transgender try to take their own lives—that's compared to approximately 1.9 percent of the general population. This figure shocks and disturbs me. I lost my brother way too early in our lives, and I *refuse* to lose my child, too. I also think of the transgender women I've met with Scott, my brother-in-law, when I've gone out with him to the bars in Hillcrest, an area in San Diego known for its acceptance of gender diversity. It devastates me to think of the sadness they keep private . . . and of the fact that my child could potentially relate to that sadness. Why shouldn't everyone just be free to live as who they are?

BRYNLEY ARRIVES ON March 31, 2012. Ryland, now four years and four months old, comes to the hospital to meet her in a T-shirt that says "Big Sis," which Jenn gave her months ago, when I first found out I was pregnant. For the past three months, Jeff and I have coached and prepped Ryland on the fact that she would need to wear it the day of Brynley's birth. I hold my breath as I hold my infant daughter, hoping that dressing Ryland wasn't a wrestle-fest for my in-laws. When the three of them arrive in the doorway of my hospital room, Ryland seems to hold back her excitement with shyness. I can see the pink hem of the Big Sis T-shirt sticking out from underneath her favorite blue sweatshirt.

As soon as she approaches Brynley, Ryland seems to forget about the shirt (and everything else). She is mesmerized with this new little being as she sits next to me on the hospital bed, staring over her sister. "What do you think, Ry?" I ask her. "Do you like her?"

Ryland nods, still taking Brynley in. She touches the pink blanket where it's swaddled around Brynley's chest, then she looks up to Jeff and says, "Can she come watch a movie with me now?"

From the very beginning, Ryland takes her job as an elder sibling very seriously and is thrilled finally to have a playmate. She is ever concerned about Brynley's well-being and security, always wondering where she is or why she's crying, and if she can hold her. I even catch Ryland crawling into Brynley's crib on multiple occasions, just to hang out, lie with her, and tell her stories. Ryland loves having this new companion to keep her company.

To be honest, I love it, too. Our house has taken on a slightly different atmosphere, with Brynley becoming a nice distraction for Ryland that focuses her away from her own struggles. Now equipped with a better understanding of what Ryland's experiences and needs are, I've become more flexible in going along with her requests . . . certainly, having an infant to care for demands that I do whatever is necessary to find the fastest solution to any particular conflict, too.

But as I stand by my child, I'm aware that I'm making a choice to stand alone. It's already clear that my in-laws are struggling to come to terms with this, and I can see that Jeff is fighting internally to know what it means, too. It's especially tricky when any friends whom we haven't seen in a while drop by to meet Brynley. In early April 2012, Matt and Michelle—who have had their hands very full with their own two small boys—come to visit. Jeff and I set up our front patio for us all to sit and catch up. When Matt and Michelle get out of their car, they're carrying gifts for all of us.

"Ryland," says Michelle, "there's a big-sister gift for you in here! Would you like to open it now?"

Ryland looks at me, and I nod. "Go on, you can open it." The present is wrapped in pink paper, and Ryland takes it hesitantly. Obediently then, she opens it. Tucked beneath the delicate pink tissue paper are sunglasses and a purse, both decorated with pretty pink-and-green watermelon slices.

Oh no.

"Ryland, what do you say to Matt and Michelle for getting you such a nice present?"

"Thank you," Ryland says politely, and puts her head down in my lap.

I want to put my head down, too—I'm so embarrassed. Here are Jeff's longtime friends, so thoughtful and generous to bring a big-sister gift that they thought would be appropriate for a little girl. "You're so welcome, honey," Michelle says sweetly, glancing at Matt, then to Jeff and me. "We hoped you would like it."

Ryland nods forcibly, her face still nestled in the skirt of my sundress. With all that she's trying to cope with, I know I can't get upset at her in front of Matt and Michelle, but I don't know what to do. I want my little girl to be appreciative of the gifts that the people we love give to her, but I'm stuck always trying to smooth things over for her. I feel like a failure because my child isn't "normal" by everyone else's standard. It's like I can't make her fit in with all of our friends' kids, and I have to constantly make excuses for why Ryland is different. The episode with Matt and Michelle makes me realize that if I want to keep this from happening again, I'll have to find a way to coach everyone on what Ryland likes.

As if *that* won't be awkward.

When Matt and Michelle leave our house, I remind Ryland how important it is to be polite and to say "thank you" when anyone presents her with a gift. I tell her that if she doesn't like what she gets, then she's allowed to tell me so later and I will return it. Then I secretly start a collection of boys' coloring books and small gifts to replace any girl-oriented gifts with something more fitting for a boy. As soon as the gift bearer leaves, I swap them swiftly, and Ryland is satisfied.

With Brynley's arrival is the further evolution of Ryland's preferences, simply because Jeff and I have less time than ever. I've finally started shopping in the boys' department for outfits I know Ryland will wear. For Easter, we all agree on a plain collared shirt, colored bright teal, to wear to the firefighter Easter egg hunt. I buy two matching bows for Ryland's hair, just to make sure everyone knows that she's a girl, and I tell myself that if we all had to compromise, at least I could dress her in pretty colors.

When we arrive at the beautiful Mission Bay Park, Ryland heads right out for the hunt and I make small talk with some of the other women, but instantly an old, familiar feeling that I've always had when I'm with the fire wives jars me: I'm never fully comfortable in my own skin with them. Everyone seems to accept that Jeff and I have a daughter who is an extreme tomboy; however, even apart from that, I've always had this very strong feeling that we don't fit in—a distance, a feeling that with Ryland's issues, I cannot truly relate to any of them. Their husbands are all very outspokenly male; the wives are confident in both themselves and their children. I feel like their lives are so simple and carefree, and we've been struggling with the complexities of navigating through Ryland's journey. As I watch Ryland hunting separately from the other children for plastic eggs filled with candy and prizes, I feel a disconnect widening between us and the families of Jeff's colleagues. As the Easter egg hunt draws to a close, all I want is to go hide in our house, where no one can ask questions or get to know what true pain and challenges are going on inside our home.

As I observe this among the adults, more and more I begin to see Ryland experiencing it with children, too. In the afternoons or evenings, I often push Bryn in the stroller and walk with Ryland to the local elementary school, where she loves to ride her scooter around the park. She always seeks out the group of older boys who live in our neighborhood and seems happy just to be in their presence, but I can feel how much she longs to be a part of their crowd. She's always the outsider, on her pink scooter with her long, blond hair flying out from underneath her blue helmet. She follows them around endlessly, and endlessly, they leave her in their dust.

I begin to decline most invitations to hang out with our neighbors because, for multiple reasons, Ryland doesn't fit in with their kids. I feel depressed and isolated for my little girl. I know she will always be different because of her ears, but to see a child left out of the crowd already, at such a young age, absolutely deflates a mother's heart.

If our circle of friends has to shrink in order for me to raise Ryland in love, then so be it. In turn, I hold on intensely to the people closest to us.

In May 2012, when Ryland is almost four and a half, my cousin Melissa graduates from nursing school. We drive up to Riverside to see her walk on graduation day. During the ceremony, while Melissa is seated with all of her classmates, her boyfriend, Andrew, tells me that he's going to propose to her. "Will you help me plan it?" he asks me. "I really want to surprise her."

I agree enthusiastically, so touched be part of such a special time in the life of the relative whom I have often considered to be as close as a sister. In July, I make up a story to lure her to the park that overlooks the beautiful Pacific Beach and Mission Bay. Andrew hires a guitarist and asks Melissa to marry him, while our family stands by watching with a video camera. After Andrew gets down on one knee and slips the ring onto her finger, Melissa cries, tells him "Yes," and hugs him . . . then instantly she comes to hug me. "Thank you for being part of this," she tells me.

"I'm so happy for you," I tell her. "Your dream is coming true."

I'm alongside her in the months to follow as she makes wedding plans, and thrilled when she asks me to be her matron of honor. I tease her and tell her there's only one condition: she has to help me plan Ryland's fifth birthday party.

"Deal," she says. "You know I'd do anything for Ryland."

Chapter Seven

Canvas for a Cause

In August 2012, Ryland shows up the first day of transitional kindergarten—a grade in some California schools that's meant to bridge the preschool experience to all-day kindergarten—wearing boys' clothes with a yellow bow in her hair. As if Ryland doesn't already stand out enough, what makes things harder is that she's constantly in the office for speech therapy, a potty accident, or early dismissal because of a hearing appointment. Also, the district audiologist and her assistant regularly come to Ryland's school to check her cochlear implants. People notice her. She's different, and she has noticeable devices that set her apart from the other children.

The first week, her teacher, Mrs. Sayers, gives me a subtle smile when she observes my face as Ryland exits the school. My daughter has learned to cope with the fashion dilemmas we're facing by zipping her jacket all the way up if she doesn't feel that her outfit is masculine enough.

That October, however, her Halloween costume is plenty masculine: Ryland wants to be Iron Man. Jenn and her in-laws host us for a trick-or-treating pre-party with chili dogs and plenty of candy. As we make our way around their neighborhood gathering treats, we meet a little boy who also is dressed as Iron Man. "What's your name?" Ryland asks him.

"It's Rylan."

Ryland looks up at me: it's her very same name without a "D" at the end, and it's her realization that if she were a boy, she could still be called Ryland.

Looking for ways to evolve Ryland's interests in a way that stays in line with who she is, Jeff and I register her for the Purple Panthers—a little girls' soccer team in our area. Because he and I both like the sport, and because we want to make sure Ryland learns the game from someone who is sensitive to her issues with hearing, we both also volunteer to be assistant coaches. Often, I chat with the other moms while sitting on a big beach blanket with Brynley, but when Jeff has to work a fire shift, I jump in and take his place.

Ryland dreads the uniform with a special passion, but Jeff has a conversation with Ryland about how we cannot choose the color of the soccer uniforms, and her team may be assigned pink or purple. Ryland reluctantly accepts this possibility, and Jeff also finds a way to make her feel more on board: he says that whatever the team's color is, he will buy a shirt to match it. As soon as the head coach informs us that the team will be called the Purple Panthers, Jeff goes to a sporting goods store and buys a purple workout shirt to wear every Saturday, which succeeds in making Ryland a little more willing.

That December, Melissa helps me plan an over-the-top fifth birthday party with a *Willy Wonka and the Chocolate Factory* theme (which I have determined is boy-oriented enough for Ryland but will appeal to kids of both genders). Melissa and I spend our time together crafting oversize Wonka bars, and colorful balloon lollipops. She borrows her mom's chocolate fondue fountain as the perfect finishing touch.

By this time I've confided in most of our friends that Ryland is a tomboy, and I make sure that everyone we invite is someone who knows that Ryland prefers "boy things," but, just to be safe, we arrange for Ryland to open her gifts after her guests have left. She's thrilled to receive mostly masculine gifts, except for one girl's shirt presented by one of our neighbors, which, all things considered, isn't too bad at all.

With the holiday planning, birthday party planning, wedding planning, and two little ones to take care of, when Jeff gets a weekend off in December, Melissa is the first person to offer to babysit Ryland and Brynley overnight so that Jeff and I can take a trip together. For a couple of days after she offers, I hesitate, thinking of how much Ryland needs me—not to mention the fact that Brynley is only nine months old and still nursing. I'm also not quite sure how to deal with the fact that Melissa has asked Ryland to be her flower girl in her wedding. When she brought it up one day with us, she tried to coax Ryland into saying she would wear a dress. I'm avoiding the conversation as much as possible because I know it's a real source of anxiety for Ry.

But I remember that my husband needs my attention, too, and how at the heart of our family is our marriage. We agree to take Melissa up on her offer, and we make a plan to travel to Las Vegas right after Christmas.

The trip's timing falls at a point when we particularly need to get away together: Ryland's issues have hit the fan.

In December 2012, I'm in our office preparing to get our holiday cards out in time for the season. Jeff is at work, Brynley is napping, and Ryland is seated beside me in the office, playing Starfall on the computer, choosing the boy-gendered character, as usual.

She glances over to see what I'm up to as I pull the cellophane wrap off the labels and the cards, delighted that they've turned out so adorably. I start to make piles—cards, envelopes, labels—for an easy assembly line of signing, stuffing, and stamping.

Ryland walks over and glances down at the Christmas card. The professional photograph on the front displays a print of Ryland and Brynley. Ryland is wearing a leopard fedora hat with a matching tie and vest, while Brynley is dressed in a matching leopard print jacket (originally a present from Macie that was intended for Ryland a few years ago).

Then Ryland picks up one of the return address labels. "Are your hands clean, honey?" I ask her.

"Yes," she says. She examines one, fully interested. Lined up on the flap of the envelope are faces of our family, emulated with little cartoon characters dressed in a festive spirit that speaks to each of our personalities. There's a man wearing a Santa hat to represent Jeff, a character with long, light brown hair and reindeer horns for me, a long-blond-haired girl with a cowboy hat for Ry, a baby with a bow on her head for Bryn, and a tan dog—Kobe. Below that appears our return address.

"Mom," Ryland says angrily, "how could you do that to me?!"
I look down at my five-year-old. "Do *what* to you?!"
"Make me look like that?!"
"Like what?"
"Like a girl!"

I set down my pen. "Ryland—what do you mean? I gave you long blond hair because you have long blond hair, and I gave you a cowboy hat because you love cowboy hats!"

Ryland's eyes begin to fill with tears. I see her bottom lip get tight as she holds back her pain.

"How should I make you look for next time?" I say, scrounging for a fix, trying to mend what is already shattered. I am so dumbfounded. What do I do or say in this moment? I know Ryland is in pain, and I'm struggling to figure out how to help my baby. It's such a lonely feeling when you know there is something your child is struggling with but you don't know how to help them. As parents, we all want to see our children grow and prosper as happy kids, then as well-adjusted teens and self-sufficient adults. We do our best to guide and teach our children when they're young, so that they will learn to be self sufficient, disciplined contributors to society who know how to deal with their own unique emotions. I think of my parents, and how they could probably understand what I'm going through; how they tried so hard to help my brother with his drug addiction. They could never seem to do enough, and I know how much pain that knowledge brought them even before the final outcome, when we lost him. The thought of this overwhelms me with fear about the same for my child.

Ryland doesn't say much until later that night. She's with me in my bedroom, where we usually read books and fall asleep together on nights when Jeff is working fire. I love to cuddle with her while Jeff is away, and I know it must be even harder for a deaf child to find comfort alone in a dark room. We remove the external portion of her implants when she sleeps, leaving her in complete silence and darkness. Knowing how frightening this may be, I have a soft spot when it comes to Ryland sleeping in our bed.

Before we take out the external implants, she lies on her tummy while I scratch her back lightly—one of her favorite things in the world. "Mom," she says. "When is Daddy coming home?"

"He'll be home tomorrow morning."

"Okay," she says. "What are we doing tomorrow?"

"You have school, and then . . ." Here, I pause. I can tell Ryland is thinking about what to say next.

"Mom . . ." she says. She wiggles away from me and sits up. Suddenly her voice is quivering. "Can I ask you something?"

"Sure, Ry. What's wrong, honey?"

"Mom, when the family dies . . . can I cut my hair so I can be a boy?"

My heart drops. Time stops. I look at her, but she is staring ahead—my stoic little child—waiting for my answer. By the expression on her face, I can see that she understands the significance of what she's just asked me. But why should we have to *die* for Ryland to cut her hair and feel happy, whatever that requires?

I don't know how to respond. I feel like I'm standing on the edge of a cliff. This is the moment when I have to choose between Ryland's happiness and being a "normal" family. I've seen and read enough to know what's coming next: this is going to shake my marriage. While I have been reading Ryland's behaviors very closely between the lines, Jeff has at times suggested that I've been "jumping to conclusions." For him, it would be ideal if Ryland were to come out and say, "Dad, you and I need to have a talk. There's something I need to share with you: I am transgender." But even if they had the cognitive capacity to do so, most five-year-olds would never initiate a serious conversation about their gender identity. No matter how many signs Ryland has shown us, it's been up to me to raise the issue.

I always feel Jeff's tension—even after their Christmas clothing shopping trip, he's avoided talking about it at all costs. Having to fathom Ryland's future as a deaf person was painful enough for Jeff, but now, dealing with yet another challenge, he has struggled, often in silence, to understand what's going on. Worse, he and I definitely have not seen the urgency of this situation in the same way.

But on this night, when Ryland breaks down, I am physically unable to see my child hurt with shame and guilt anymore. I can no longer allow this to go on. I have to choose. The reality of all this has been creeping up on me for some time, but as a mother, my first priority has to be my child's safety.

"Ryland . . . honey . . . " I sit up in bed. "You don't have to wait until the family dies. You can get your hair cut right now."

She begins to cry again. Her tears are silent, her face is flushed. She seems to know that her pain is hurting me, too, and neither of us knows how to make it all stop.

Even at this tiny age, Ryland has the wisdom and self-awareness to know the true significance of what she has just asked me. Cutting her hair is the final bridge left to cross into letting her become a boy. If that makes my child like herself better, then I'm prepared to do it.

I wrap my arms around her. She removes her ears and hands them to me—her signal that she's finished having a conversation and is ready to rest. She buries her head into the space under my arm, and she cries. I massage her head and her back until I know she's fallen asleep.

And then I begin my own cries. My child, only five years old, is so miserable with who she is. For months I have seen a conversation like this coming. It pains me to think that this little person is smart enough to tell me something so powerful, at such a young age. These tears are for my child—my desire to make things right for Ryland. The final and complete acceptance that this is not a phase, that this isn't just going to pass, that my daughter isn't just a tomboy. That on the other side of all this, things will be different—Ryland's life, Jeff's life, Brynley's life—our family will be changed.

My tears flow harder when I begin to visualize Ryland's future as a transgender person. Just like I had pictured Ryland sitting at the Thanksgiving table without sound, I begin to picture her as a teenager not having a date to prom because she is the "different" one.

And many of my tears are disbelief that this is really happening. *How could God do this to us again? How could he put this little person through so much in life—what was He trying to do to us?* I'm angry that God would make this innocent little child hurt so much inside. Then I think, *How am I going to explain this to everyone? How will I deal with Jeff? How will I get everyone to understand that I didn't do this to my child?*

My mind races with thoughts. I begin to anticipate the comments from the naysayers already, and to practice my responses. I can't let this go on. I have to get to the bottom of what is going on inside Ryland, and I have to fix my child's pain. I have to take action.

The next morning, I'm in Ryland's bedroom, choosing her outfit for school . . . and hoping that when she wakes up, she'll have forgotten about the terrible conversation we had last night.

Without skipping a beat, I'm pulling out underwear and socks when I look to her doorway and find her staring at me.

"Mom?" she says.

"What is it, Ry?"

"Why did God make me this way?"

What?

All over again, I'm at a loss. Completely. I search for the words, the thought, to spin this into something positive. "What do you mean, baby?"

She rubs one foot against the opposite ankle with an innocence that strikes at my heart. Then she leans back against the doorway. "Why didn't God make me a boy?"

I have no idea what to say or do, so I take the response that comes to me automatically. I walk to my tiny child, I put my arms around her, and I squeeze her in to me. We stay this way for a few moments, and silently, I make my vow. *Ryland,* I think, *even if one day this means that we have to leave Daddy and our family so that you can be free with me from the judgment of anyone who doesn't accept you, then I will do what I have to do.* My pain and anguish are starting to turn to anger—and anger, I've heard, is the powerful agent that catalyzes us to make critical changes in our lives.

I prepare Ryland for school. As always, I time everything precisely: change Brynley's diaper, feed both children, make a lunch, load them up, and get to school early enough to grab a decent parking spot—the perfect flow of the morning's timing that is crucial to most moms.

I drop Ryland off, but I don't know if it's the right thing to do. I feel very reluctant to release my little one into the classroom, into the world, into her day of thinking and interacting and learning, when there's no way for me to influence what she'll experience. I make sure Ryland has her snack separate from her lunch on the lunch cart and her FM system turned on and placed around her neck in order to pick up the teacher's voice directly. Then, when it's eight o'clock, we hear the bell ring.

I walk with Ryland to the line outside of her class, where I kiss her good-bye. Mrs. Sayers greets each student with a hug when they enter her classroom. As I watch Ryland go inside, my heart feels a tug as painful as it did on the very first day I ever dropped her off at school. *Is my child going to be okay today?*

Before I pull out of the school parking lot, I text my mom and ask her to find all the old photos of me as a little girl during my pixie haircut phase. I used to hate those pictures, but I want to relate to Ryland somehow, any way I can, so that she won't feel so alone.

When we arrive home, I sit Brynley onto her blanket on the living room floor and stand there thinking, reflecting, in the way one does when everything in their life has just shifted.

Then suddenly, a memory rises up.

It was an afternoon late last summer when I was feeling very alone, very lost and sad, pondering the fact that Ryland was less than a month away from entering transitional kindergarten with so many battles happening inside of her. At that time, I was under the deepest impression that she was showing me signs that she was a lesbian. It's when things were growing clear to me that this wasn't a phase, or something she would outgrow—I just felt it.

That day, Peg and Rand had the kids so that I could get some errands done. I craved the feeling of being surrounded by other people . . . but I didn't want to have to speak to any of them. And I wanted to see something beautiful. I took the impulse to drive to Mission Valley's outdoor mall with its palm trees rising up like pillars and its sleek, bright construction.

The only thing I had any intention to buy was an Orange Julius and an order of mini pretzels with warm cheese sauce. For a few minutes, I sat on the bench and enjoyed every morsel, every sip. Pure pleasure . . . it was a contentment that I hadn't experienced in as long as I could remember.

Just as I stood up to wander a little more, a middle-aged woman approached me. For some reason, I remember that I found myself not immediately inclined to dismiss her. Her clipboard had some paperwork on it, and when I glanced down, I saw the image of a rainbow on the paper. "Do you have a few minutes?" she said. Ryland and Brynley were taken care of. What would a few more minutes be, if it had any potential to lead me to some clarity?

"Yes," I told her. "I have a minute or two."

She shared a very emotional story about a young woman who came out as a lesbian and was not accepted by her family. She grew visibly emotional as she told it, and suddenly I was so glad that I'd given her the chance to speak. She asked me whether I'd like to donate to the nonprofit she was representing, whose main goal was to raise awareness about the experiences of the LGBTQ population.

"I will absolutely donate," I told her, and I couldn't stop myself from asking: "Can I tell you something?"

She nodded and stood patiently. And I poured my heart out.

I told her that no one really understood what I was going through, that my husband didn't even really understand. I told her the painful stories of Ryland hiding in the closet wearing Jeff's clothes and making me promise not to tell anyone. I told her every little indication I had that my child was either lesbian or transgender. There were so many. I broke down and cried, and she hugged me, right there in the middle of the mall. I gave her a donation, and she gave me a slip of paper with the contact information for their free help line.

When I arrived at home, I tucked the paper far into one of my dresser drawers. If Jeff found it, he would probably be very angry, for two reasons: one, we were on a tight budget and he probably wouldn't have been thrilled that I was donating money without his consent, and two, he might be upset that I was "jumping to conclusions" about Ryland.

I held on to this piece of paper for a long time. I didn't do anything with it, but since I knew I was certainly no expert on this subject, something told me that it might come in handy one day. I know now that I saved that piece of paper with the same dedicated resourcefulness I used when we were researching the possibility of Ryland's cochlear implants: There had to be other families who had gone through this before us, who could give us some strength and direction to the resources we needed back then; who could enlighten us with lessons from their experiences. During that period, I didn't know if we'd be able to make it through all that—but now we have. That experience in our family's life solidified the belief for me that I can always learn from someone just by asking for help.

Now, I know I have to do the same thing in this case. I have to find every story and person I can who might relate to my child, and to help me find which path is best for our family.

Back in our living room as Brynley lifts her head and wiggles her arms to stay occupied, I pick up my phone again and quickly punch out an email. It's to Aunt Sue, Rand's sister, who is gay and has been an advocate for the LGBTQ population for many years. "Call me if you can," I write. "Ryland just shocked me with a comment. I need an honest opinion. xoxo."

A minute later, I jump when I see her name in my inbox, but it's an automatic reply message. She's away traveling on business and will respond to emails when she returns to California.

Then, remembering the slip of paper with rainbows on it from Canvas for the Cause, I dash back to my bedroom and fumble into the back of my drawer. Yes! There it is. I run back to the living room and quickly dial the number.

"Hello, this is Shannon," says a friendly voice.

"Hi," I tell her. "Ummm . . . my name is Hillary, and I met one of your activists months ago at Mission Valley. I've been wanting to call you for months, but I haven't."

"I'm glad you did," Shannon says. "What's the reason for your call?"

I take a deep breath and launch into it. "My daughter has been showing signs of being gay. She's five. She dresses in my husband's clothes and only wants to do boy things. But recently, it's gotten more serious. The other night she said to me, 'Mom, when the family dies, I'm going to cut my hair so I can be a boy.' Then this morning she looked at me with tears in her eyes and asked why God made her this way. I am at the point that I don't know what to say to her. I really don't. I am okay with her being a lesbian, but I just don't think that is it."

Shannon's voice is consistently calm and kind. "I can find you some help," she says. "We'll get you some support groups and resources in your area. If you're open to my honest opinion—"

"I am."

"It sounds to me like Ryland may be transgender."

The word actually gives me a sense of relief—finally, someone has validated what I've been guessing. "What do I do?"

"Maybe you can start referring to Ryland as 'them' or 'they.'"

I try to turn this phrase over in my head, but my thoughts are on spin cycle.

"Here," Shannon says. "I'm going to give you the names of a few therapists Ryland could see. You and your husband should go, as well. Most of the ones I know are for ages fourteen and above, but I will call around and do some research to make sure we can find someone who's appropriate for you."

"I'll appreciate absolutely any resources you have," I tell her. "I'll do whatever you suggest." When we hang up, that moment of relief is short-lived. More than ever, this is very real . . . and the area underneath my rib cage is sick with emotion. I'm worried for Ryland's future.

Shannon calls me later that day, before Ryland gets out of school. "I have two names for you to contact," she says. "These are both very good therapists who deal with gender identity." One is Marcie Goldman, and the other is Darlene Tando. In addition, she's called both of them and left messages on our behalf. She also tells me about an underground parent support group in San Diego that meets every month, and she offers to put me in touch with the group leader.

Ryland and Brynley are both in bed when Jeff comes home that night. I ask him to sit down with me, and I tell him what Ryland told me the night before. Pushing against my own tears to try to keep from breaking down, I also observe Jeff's reaction: the conversation is definitely bringing him farther down the path to acceptance and the need to explore more of what Ryland is experiencing.

"Honey," I tell him, feeling my affection for him bubbling up again now that I'm seeing the authenticity in his reaction. "I know how hard this is for you—and I know I handle it differently, but trust me, this is *not* any easier for me."

He looks at me, waiting patiently to hear what's coming next.

"But staying in denial is not going to make this go away. We need to talk to other parents—some who can offer some guidance for how we could be handling this."

After a silent pause, Jeff nods. "Okay," he says. "Let's see if we can find any resources." We walk into the office, where he sits down at the computer. "What should we search for?" he says.

"Start with 'transgender kids.'"

Up comes the name of a transgender girl, Jazz Jennings, whose name I've come across every time I've done a search on the topic. I urge Jeff to click on a video of her on a recent talk show, and I raise my eyebrows at him when he sees how confident she is in the interview. "Wow," he says. "She's so happy."

There's also a list of a few books by experts, so I order every book I can find on the topic of gender nonconformity, like *The Transgender Child* by Stephanie Brill and Rachel Pepper. When it arrives three days later, I break down crying as I read. It's a huge "aha" moment when *The Transgender Child* lists the four distinguishing characteristics that can indicate that a child is indeed transgender: bathroom behavior, swimsuit aversion, their underwear preferences, and the type of toys they choose. Ryland meets all four.

In this moment, I am officially convinced.

The very next day, Ryland and Brynley are in the bath together, and knowing now what we're dealing with, I videotape it with my phone. When I hit the RECORD button, Ryland puts her arm around Brynley and says, "This is my sister Brynley, and I'm her brudder, Ryland."

Immediately I hit the STOP button, as if out of reflex. Then I take a deep breath and send the video to Jeff at work. My subject line reads one word: "wow."

The statement is clear and simple.

Part Two

Embracing Our Son

Chapter Eight

Transitional Kindergarten

Christmas is a temporary reprieve when my parents—er, Santa—present Ryland with an amazing battery-powered kids' quad vehicle. As Jeff assembles it in our garage, Peg comes out to join him. From the kitchen I can overhear her when she says, "You know, I've been reading that book that Hillary gave me, called *The Transgender Child*. Maybe there's really something to this with Ryland, Jeff. What do you think?"

"I don't know, Mom," he says. "I'll wait for Ryland to tell me." I shake my head to myself and continue my work in the kitchen, knowing he still can't look this situation as squarely in the face as I've come to do.

On Christmas Day, Ryland rides the quad around our property with such authority that the neighbor boys, usually so oblivious to her presence, stand at our fence and gaze at her in wonder. Two days later, Chase's grandma, with whom I shared our latest updates before school let out for the holiday break, emails me with a suggestion to read a book called *Raising My Rainbow*, about a woman's gender-nonconforming son, named CJ. Immediately I order it and thank Barbara for the recommendation. Her validation has been such a source of strength, and her overwhelming support has given me a sense of comfort and security at a time when I've been in such desperate need for people to understand what we're going through.

The night before New Year's Eve, when we know most couples are putting the finishing touches on their party plans, Jeff and I are discussing Ryland. The topic is feeling much easier for me to bring up, and finally I'm starting to feel like I have a teammate in Jeff.

"I wonder if there's any kind of network in this area of families with transgender children," I tell him. "Wouldn't it be perfect if we could find something like the group we had after the cochlear implants?" Jeff sits down at the computer, and he begins to search for resources online to find out if there are any kind of support groups in Southern California for transgender children and their families.

"Shift Happens," Jeff says.

"Huh?" I lean in over his shoulder to see the website he's pulled up—it's a parent support group in Orange County started by Sarah Tyler. "Hey, I remember her!" I tell Jeff. "I've seen her on TV."

Sarah Tyler is the mom of two beautiful children and the wife of an Orange County police officer. Her seven-year-old child tried to run into oncoming traffic because Sarah wouldn't allow him to wear a princess dress for Halloween. On the TV interview, she discussed how she and her husband had embraced their son's transition to be female. I found their story extremely inspiring.

Jeff sends a request to the website's contact-us section, and that evening the phone rings. On the line is Sarah herself. She is friendly, she's soothing, and she promises that she's going to get us to the next right place. It's the first telephone conversation with another mom in months that brings me to laugh. Our families share so many common experiences.

"If your husband works nights," she says, "I know what that's like. Please don't hesitate to call me for some company, anytime."

In the meantime, Shannon puts me in touch with Monica, who's the leader of the San Diego Transforming Family support group. When I call Monica, I can tell that she's a woman who touches everyone she meets. Her son, Isaac, was one of the first kids to openly transition in the San Diego area, during a time when this subject was met with great hostility and misunderstanding. When Monica tells me that Isaac is pursuing his education at Stanford University, I know this will help Jeff see that this is the kind of kid we want to serve as an inspiration for Ryland. Having fully entered the acceptance phase of this, my natural inclination has been to seek out positive people who are dealing with this same thing in their families. If Jeff begins to see that Ryland can be happy, normal, and successful while being transgender, I'm hopeful that it will continue to evolve his thinking about Ryland's situation.

Recognizing a need in our area, Monica started the support group along with a middle-aged transgender man named Connor. From what Monica explains, they've grown significantly over the past few years as parents are beginning to listen to their children. Their first meeting for the year will take place the first week in January. Jeff agrees to go with me in an effort to start our new year with as much calm in our home as we can.

Peg and Rand respond enthusiastically when we ask them to

babysit that night. We tell Ryland nothing about the meeting; we ourselves have no idea what to expect, or if we'll ever return for a second meeting. For the safety of the children, the San Diego Transforming Family support group is completely underground. It's not advertised on the LGBT center website, and you can't find any information about it online.

Monica directs us to where it's located. When we enter the meeting place, we find the parents sitting separately from the children while the kids go to a supervised playroom in another part of the building. Jeff and I exchange a look, aware that this makes sense: they separate the adults from their children so the parents can talk openly about their struggles.

As the meeting starts, it seems gentle enough, but I can't help but feel scared out of my mind. Everyone sits in a circle and takes a turn introducing themselves and stating pieces of their child's story.

Seated next to me is a younger man wearing a fedora hat, like Ryland's. When I meet his eyes, he flashes me a warm smile. Nervously, I smile back. On the other side of him sits a woman who's about my age. As the sharing circle nears our turn, I'm so anxious, I believe everyone can probably see my pulse throbbing through my neck. On the way here, Jeff and I agreed that we didn't really want to tell everyone our story. "I don't really feel like pouring my heart out and telling our story to a bunch of strangers," he said.

"I know, that's what I'm nervous about, too," I told him. "But let's just hear what the parents have to say."

"I know, it can't hurt us to go and listen. I'm sure we can learn from their experiences. I just don't want to say a lot." For him, it's still too personal, and for me, I know I'll cry. I'm so fragile and ready to crack wide open from being forced to stifle these emotions for so long. But with everyone else sharing so openly, for Jeff and me to pass on our chance to speak would draw as much attention as if we were to spill a puddle from our hearts into the middle of the circle.

As I listen to the other families share their stories, immediately it's clear to me that our child is the youngest in the group. When it's my turn, I follow their format: I share Ryland's name, gender, and how long she has been trying to express herself as a boy. Seated a few parents down from me is another mom whose now-daughter is transgender and, she says, just a little bit older than Ryland. She says that for a long time, her husband still tried to buy his daughter little-boy socks and clothes. She was already presenting as a girl and going to school as a female, but the woman's husband has struggled very hard as the little girl's father—by the sounds of it, even harder than Jeff has.

In this first meeting, we learn that this is actually typical: the father of the transgender child usually experiences a great deal more turmoil about accepting his transgender child than the mother does. I relate, and I develop my own theories for why this is: perhaps it has something to do with a mother's empathy and intuition, or maybe it's that the mom usually spends more time with her children than the dad does and so is more attuned to what the children are experiencing. The woman shares that it seems as though finally her husband may be coming on board, and she breaks into billowing sobs when she turns to us and says, "I'm just so happy to see another family here with a child the same age as mine, and you are so lucky to have your husband here." I look at Jeff, who's listening intently from where he's seated next to me. I take his hand. Not one day of this has been easy, but this woman is right: I *am* lucky. Jeff was willing to listen and learn with me this first time, together.

Later on, another parent begins to explain the grief and suffering that she and her child are going through with insurance and medical professionals. Insurance won't pay for hormone blockers or cross hormones. Many hormone blockers cost around twenty thousand dollars per treatment, with treatments needed three to four times a year. Many insurance companies will not pay for "top" surgery until a child is on testosterone for at least a year, but many teens cannot get a doctor to prescribe testosterone because the teen is depressed. There are so many twists and turns to navigate, and the insurance companies really don't have a human appreciation for what children and families go through with this. "Maybe things will change soon," the mother says, and sighs. "We just have to wait and see."

My hands clench around the edge of my seat. *Wait for what?! I want to ask her. You have to DO something! You can't just sit around and wait for everyone else to do it! WE have to fight, we're the parents! Who will do it better than we will? Who will do it at all?*

Unlike me, Jeff remains calm, if visibly disturbed, as he listens to the other parents tell their stories—always harrowing, sometimes horrible. There are multiple accounts about teenagers who absolutely despise their bodies so brutally that many of them refuse to bathe because of their self-disgust. Others bind their chests so tightly to hide their breasts after puberty that they've collapsed a lung or gotten severe skin infections. Nearly every single one of the parents talks about their children's struggles with their peers at school and often even their teachers.

And all of the parents in the room share one common theme: they all wish they would have transitioned their teenagers much sooner in their lives. The onset of puberty has multiplied their problems. Once puberty hits, there are some irreversible changes that cause many transgender preteens and teens to experience major discomfort, sadness, withdrawal, and thoughts of suicide.

Something clicks: this is all Jeff needs to hear. On the ride home, he begins to open up and share some of his thoughts with me.

"As reluctant as I was," he says, "I'm glad we went."

"You are?"

"Yeah. Those stories were heartbreaking. I get the consequences we're facing if we don't address more of what's going on. I don't ever want to see Ryland go through those struggles. I'm on the same page now, Hill. I get it."

As the words leave his mouth, I can tell, really, that he's finally got it. We do not want Ryland to fall into this hugely depressed, self-destructing group of children who are suffering to be who they are. Despite the overwhelming emotions that I just experienced during the meeting, I am overcome with joy as I hear Jeff speaking. I know that we are now on the same page, standing side by side on this journey. Jeff has always been a source of strength for me, and together we've overcome some of life's biggest challenges and struggles. It had pained me to feel like I was on this journey alone for so long, and now, in this moment, I know that I have my partner by my side.

The following week, Jeff and I drive with Ryland to Hillcrest for our first appointment with Darlene Tando. Her entrance requires inputting a private code, to ensure clients' safety, and inside, the office atmosphere is quaint and comfortable. As we take a seat in the small waiting room, I point out to Jeff the white noise machine that she keeps in her hallway to guarantee that the conversation happening inside her office is sacred and confidential.

My heart beats with the same fear I felt the week before at the Transforming Family support group meeting. Among all the emotions bubbling up in me is frustration: during one of our conversations about Ryland, Jeff stated that he thinks it makes the most sense for us to wait until Ryland starts actual kindergarten, which is another five months away, before we begin the transition. I *do* see his point—it's a lot for us to hope that Ryland's tiny classmates would understand when they're reintroduced to Ryland in the new gender—but after the support group meeting last week, I feel a stark sense of urgency about this. In my mind, the sooner we allow Ry to do this, the better.

Darlene's demeanor instantly helps to calm me. She has a wide, beautiful smile and an air of kindness and authority over her work. When she tells us that she herself has small children, I observe Jeff ease up a bit, too. For the first time, we both feel more understood and not so alone. We tell her all about Ryland's history, including her persistent and consistent cross-gender identification, her insistence that she is a boy, and her most recent comment about wanting to cut her hair after the family dies. After getting this extensive history from Jeff and me, Darlene requests to spend some time alone getting to know Ryland, so she can ask her questions and Ryland can respond without our parental influence and her desire to please us. During her assessment, she asks Ryland how she would like to be addressed, to which Ryland responds confidently and swiftly: "Please call me a boy."

With her evaluation complete, we reconvene with Darlene. Her time with Ryland confirms what we already know: Ryland has the heart and brain of a boy.

When she brings Jeff and me back in, Darlene affirms my thinking. "The longer you wait to transition a child, the more emotional damage you may cause," she says. "My recommendation, based on all of the things you've told me, is that you need to try using male pronouns immediately and socially transition Ryland as soon as possible."

Jeff looks at me with hesitation. We had a feeling that this was coming. He chimes in. "What if we were to wait a few months until the school year is over?"

"I understand that this is a very big 'decision,' if you will, for any parent to make about a child," Darlene says. "I don't always recommend transition the first time I meet with parents—it depends on where they are in the process of acceptance and how resistant they are. But from everything I've heard today, it sounds like the two of you have already come to a lot of conclusions on your own—am I right?"

Jeff and I look at each other and nod. "Yes," I tell her.

"I want to encourage you to continue to do all the research you still feel is necessary to move forward from here. Ultimately, how you handle this has to be your choice."

"If you were us," I ask her, "what would you do?"

She nods, as if she was anticipating that question, and this makes me feel validated for having asked. "From everything that the two of you and Ryland have shared with me today, I believe continuing to force a child to live in such an uncomfortable state, even for a few months, could be even more detrimental than making an awkward transition mid-school year."

After giving it a second's thought, Jeff looks at me. He nods. We're both convinced now that this transition needs to happen sooner rather than later. I find myself tearing up as I tell Darlene,

"In my heart and my gut, I've known the truth about Ryland. We just needed a professional to back us up and confirm what we already knew was best."

"I completely get that," she says. "And if you'd like, I can begin to guide you in how to begin the transition—how does that sound?"

"Yes, please," Jeff says, as I dab the corners of my eyes to catch my tears. "That would be great."

With an approach that is equal parts straightforward and gentle, Darlene starts to use pronouns that refer to Ryland as a male—*he, him,* and *his,* instead of *she, her,* and *hers.* At first I silently cringe at the thought of getting used to this, but slowly, cautiously, we begin to follow suit to adopt the male pronouns. In this environment, led by a professional, there's enough room for adjustment not to hurt Ryland's feelings.

It is extremely awkward at first. It's like a foreign language—and without even looking at him, I know that Jeff feels similarly. Darlene explains that as challenging as this may be for us, other people will follow our lead in referring to Ryland as a boy. When they slip up and refer to Ryland as "she," it will be up to us to correct them.

At the end of the appointment, she tells us, "I know how difficult this part of the journey can be, but look at you two, already correcting yourselves. It's very impressive!"

Jeff and I exchange a humble smile, relieved to be feeling like we're doing the right thing for Ryland. Darlene sends us off with the recommendation to arrange meetings with Ryland's teacher, principal, speech therapist, and school psychologist, which I do as soon as we get home. I also send an email to Jenn, Gianna's mom, to share the status of all that's been going on. *It has been a whirlwind around here,* I tell her. *We have finally figured out that Ryland is a transgender boy.* As soon as I type it, I acknowledge the certainty of it for the first time, and it's as though I have released an unwieldy balloon into the sky. The truth is out. The truth will set us free.

But first, it will test our strength.

ON JANUARY 15, 2013, we decide to execute the task that will be the first step in the official transition and that may evolve everything at turbo speed: getting Ryland's hair cut. We just don't quite know how to go about it.

This will be a pivotal experience in Ryland's life, and Jeff doesn't want to cause a stir at his barbershop down the street, with its staff of very devout Catholic men who speak mostly Spanish. I understand, but I can sense that this is his way of cowering and it upsets me. "Why don't I just cut it!" I tell him one night, fresh out of patience. I turn to Ryland. "Ry, do you want me to cut your hair?"

Ryland's eyes light up.

"Hill, wait—don't you think we should have it done professionally?"

"Well, you won't take her—I mean him—down to your barber." We have begun to correct ourselves on pronouns . . . constantly.

"Okay," he says, "fine. Maybe just a little. What if we just do a shorter girl's cut to start?"

I shrug, exasperated.

"Ryland," Jeff says, "come sit down. Mom's going to cut your hair." Ryland looks at us both with wide eyes, his hopes about to come true. "But there's something we need to explain first. Some people may not understand why you've cut your hair, okay? And you'll just have to tell them you like it shorter."

Ryland looks up at me and I ask him, "Are you sure you want to do this, honey?"

Ry nods.

I gently pull Ryland's long, beautiful, blond hair into a ponytail, past his cochlear receivers, which are colored with adhesive "skins" that are decorated with characters from his favorite cartoon: *Power Rangers.* I take a deep breath—his hair is like corn silk in my palm. Then, very carefully, I begin to snip across the hair that falls immediately above the nape of his neck. The snips are taking effort, which prolongs the process and makes me even more emotional. This could be the last time I ever see my child with long hair. It feels monumental, but so scary at the same time.

Then, suddenly, Ryland breaks down. Jeff and I look at each other in confusion as he wails with loud, hysterical sobs. "What is it, honey?"

He begins to shake uncontrollably and cry. "No!" he says. "Put it back on! Put it back on!" Our child stands with his back to me, hysterical, now with hair that is just below his ear on the right and shoulder length on the left.

"I can't leave it like this!" I tell Jeff.

"Honey," Jeff says. "We thought you would be so happy to have your hair cut short; wasn't this what you wanted?"

Ryland is sobbing so hard that he can't communicate what's going on. Eventually we convince him to let me finish the cutting job, telling him that it's not too horribly short. But it's not until we see Darlene Tando the following week that we understand what actually happened.

We didn't realize it at the time, but we pushed our fears for what others would think onto Ryland when Jeff warned him that people might not understand it. We were trying to protect Ryland by forewarning him of people's judgments; trying to help him anticipate what people might say and strategize how he could explain the haircut—but instead of setting him up to win, our idea just confirmed that he should be worried about what other people think of him. We alerted him to fear rejection from his classmates, and we made it his job to defend his reason for doing it. Now, with Darlene's insight, we understand: that was supposed to be our job. "So we should have said something like, 'Ryland, you will look so handsome with short hair! You are going to rock short hair!'"

Darlene gives us a forgiving wince. "Well, yes," she says. "That might have been a better approach." Instead, we warned Ryland that others may not like it or understand him. This is a moment of learning for us when Darlene explains, "It's best to avoid warning Ryland of others' opinions again. It will teach him that others' opinions are more important than his own feelings." Darlene says that we need to embrace him and support him as a boy, and only allow positive people and energy to come into our world. It's our job now to be the best protectors and the biggest fans of our child—our boy. In things I've read and in our support group, I've heard parents say that they're waiting for their child to initiate the transition—but kids are kids! They won't initiate the transition without their parents' blessing. It's our responsibility, mine and Jeff's, to establish how we expect people to treat Ryland, the boy.

Jeff takes Ryland down to a kids' salon and has his hair evened out into a cut that falls just beneath his ears. Ryland returns home beaming. I'm amazed at how everything has just changed, but my child is still absolutely beautiful.

Now, with Ryland presenting as a boy, we know that we have to address it. Imagine running into someone we know—friends of friends, one of Ryland's former teachers, someone from the cochlear implant team—who's speechless and baffled because the Ryland they knew was a little girl dressed in frills and bows. I would feel the heat of the blood start to fill my face as I struggle to find the words to explain what was going on, without also offending my now-son standing before them.

I admit this is *more* of my own fear of others' judgment, but also, it could hurt Ryland severely if they react to him negatively. I begin to *force* myself to get past this fear of judgment. I know my child's life depends on how I demonstrate courage in each scenario we face. I cannot avoid running into people who knew us before the transition—we're a familiar family in a close community. It's inevitable.

In hopes that it will alleviate much of the stress of trying to explain our five-year story to all of them, Jeff and I decide that it's necessary to write a letter and send it to everyone we know—our family, friends, neighbors, a very select few of Jeff's coworkers who know Ryland and our situation extremely well. This letter will need to answer any questions before anyone even has the opportunity to ask. I've heard so many questions already, and for the last three years we've grown exhausted of bold and uninformed comments that people have given us unsolicited: "It's a phase!" "Take the boy stuff away!" or "It's okay, she's a tomboy." No, no, no. I'm so tired of hearing everyone's opinion and questions. It's time for me to take a stand. The letter is intended to set a boundary, and I intend to stick to it.

For guidance, I refer to the book *The Transgender Child* and the website genderspectrum.com. Then, bearing in mind the things Darlene has taught us about the importance of Ryland's emotional well-being, with Jeff's help I craft the following message:

Dear Friends and Family,

This is an incredibly difficult letter to write. As you all know, Ryland was a late talker due to her Deaf diagnosis at 13 months old. But, from the moment Ryland could hear and speak—at around 20 months of age—she would scream, "I am a boy!" until she would break down into tears. We thought it was a little odd, but we laughed it off. We also thought it to be simply a phase, but this behavior has continued and strengthened over time. Our concern has led Jeff and I to seek help from numerous professionals and countless resources to help us discover the root of Ryland's consistent expression as a boy. Many of you have seen them, and there are certainly more examples than I can write, but a few of the instances that stood out are:

- Hiding in Jeff's closet so she could put his clothes on while making me promise not to tell anyone that she was a boy. Her shame was very unsettling at such a young age!
- Temper tantrums starting at age 2, whenever we made Ryland wear dresses, skirts, or female Halloween costumes. We initially thought this was her

being a spoiled brat, but later realized it was more about the pain of looking like a girl than Ryland being a defiant child.

- Self-portraits are always male.
- Only desiring typically male toys and colors.
- Refusing to wear girls' bathing suits beginning at age 2. Wanting to wear no shirt.
- Trying to stand up to urinate on multiple occasions.
- Desiring and hiding in order to wear boys' underpants (she had an accident and borrowed a pair of boys underwear at a friend's house).
- Purposefully ripping her girl hat she made at school, so she didn't have to wear it.
- Not wanting to go to fun events if she had to be a girl (in dress).
- Obsessing over and questioning gender in strangers that have gender-neutral looks.
- Always choosing to be the "dad" when playing house with friends.

Though these may seem trivial to some, the turning point came this last December when Ryland saw the return address labels I personalized for our family Christmas card. Ryland burst into tears when she saw that her personalized character had long, blond hair. She began crying, "Mom, how could you make me look like that?! You gave me long hair and made me look like a girl!" I didn't know how to respond. She continued to cry that night in bed and through the tears and a quivering lip she said to me, "Mom, when our family dies, I will cut my hair so I can be a boy." Ryland obviously did not want to disappoint us by transitioning to a boy while we (her family) were still alive. It made my heart break to think that Ryland would think she had to wait until we died to be who she really felt she was inside! The next day continued with sadness when she said, "Why did God make me this way? Why didn't He make me a boy?" Again, I didn't know how to answer my baby, but I knew I couldn't hide this pain anymore.

As mentioned above, I began reading books, watching documentaries, contacting multiple agencies, and sought as many professionals as I could find. Jeff and I have met with the leading specialists and doctors, attended support groups, talked to families with similar stories, and researched as much as possible. We have determined that Ryland is a transgender child.

Although Ryland was physically born with female anatomy, her brain is that of a boy.

Jeff and I will be the first to admit that we struggle with it sometimes—not because we are ashamed of him in any way, but because it makes us worry for his safety: we stick out; people stare and comment. The natural instinct is to blend in; no one likes to be the one everyone is whispering about! We are constantly having to weigh the importance of validating Ryland's feelings about who he is (that is, not stifling his need to do boy things) and doing everything possible to make sure that he doesn't begin to think there is something "wrong" with him. As parents of a transgender child, it's frightening to know that there is only so much we can do to protect Ryland's self-esteem from a sometime harsh and demonizing world. What we do know, however, is that living in secrecy and shame is not good for any of us.

We are providing this letter because, if it were you having issues in your family that were as important as this, we would want to understand what those issues were and be able to be informed and supportive. Along those lines, there is a lot more information out there about gender variance than I have summarized here and if you are interested we are happy to share.

Below, there are a couple of resources that you might find of interest and we can certainly share other resources if you desire to read more.

We know that if we had said nothing at all, you would accept and love Ryland just as he is. Now that we have said something, I also know that you will choose to either support or not support our decision to let Ryland live as a boy. This means we are listening to Ryland's request to present as a boy in appearance and to be referred to as he/him. If you DO decide to support us, please also support our decision to let Ryland express himself freely, decide what to wear, and present to the world as he chooses. We expect that you will love, play, discipline, and enjoy him in every way possible, and encourage him to be the happiest and best person he is capable of being. He should not get any extra slack for being different—he needs to learn from each of you how to behave like a good person and that is what we hope you will teach him.

These are the things we try to do to support Ryland, and to help him build a strong character and sense of self: We hope you, our family and friends, will help us in doing everything possible to see that he aspires to great things. For now, we just want our home and our friends' and families' homes to be his "safe" places where he can be himself. To that end, we ask you to:

- Love him for who he is.
- Validate him—whenever it comes up or there is conversation, let him know that you know it to be true that there is more than one way to be a boy or a girl, that you imagine it is hard that some kids don't get how you feel, etc.
- Encourage his individuality (you look handsome in that suit) and avoid stereotypical comments.
- Acknowledge and celebrate difference—he is different and knows it and there is nothing to be ashamed of—when he wants to talk about it, talk about it; give examples of how you are different or how being different can be great!
- Try and deal with your own judgments—recognize your own internal issues about gender and how they play in to your feelings about Ry.
- Be Ryland's advocate—if you are with him in a situation where something is awkward—someone is teasing or judgmental—speak up for him, and help him speak up for himself.
- No victim blaming—Ryland is not responsible for

other people's intolerance—neither he nor we, his family/friends, have to "accept" that people are going to be judgmental; nor does he/we have to constantly be hiding who he is in order to fit in. When people tease, bully, or are intolerant, they are the ones at fault. Not Ryland.

- Think about acceptance in other things that you do—making the world OK for Ryland means we all have to work on squashing eons of ingrained stereotypes; think of ways to line up or sort people other than "boys in one line, girls in another." Advocate for others who are different and struggling. Examine the world around you and step up/speak out when someone is treated unfairly or unjustly because they are not like you and don't blend in.

- *You also must know that if you choose to not support our decision, please don't expect our relationship to grow from here. Our child's happiness is most important to us.*

We are sure that this may be confusing for some of you. It certainly was for us at the beginning and caused us many tears and sleepless nights. What we have learned, however, is that most children realize their "true gender" between 3 to 5 years of age. This has been the case with many families we have met on similar journeys with their children. We have also learned that our child's transgender identity is not a result of our parenting style, family structure, or environmental factors and that there is nothing anyone can do to change a child's gender identity. This is not just a phase for Ryland or something that he will outgrow. All of the research has shown that therapeutic attempts to change the child into an acceptance of the born gender are both unsuccessful and detrimental to the child's mental health. Simple fixes, such as removing all of the male clothing and toys and forcing Ryland into living as a girl, were both examined and found to be full of more harm than good. Our goals for Ryland are the same as when we brought him home from the hospital: to be happy, feel good about himself, to find what he is good at, and to know that he is loved unconditionally. These goals have not changed now that we recognize Ryland's gender identity.

We are aware of the uphill journey ahead for our now son, and for our entire family, but the alternative of denying who he is puts him at a high risk of depression, anxiety, sexual acting out, substance abuse, and suicide. These are not options for us. Studies have shown that transgender people who have been raised without support for their gender identity have an attempted suicide rate of 41%, while the national average is 1.9%. We will not choose to be unsupportive of our son and hope that he will not fall into the 41%. We will do anything in our power to make sure he is part of the 59% that never attempts to take his own life. Our love and support for Ryland is complete. We hope yours will be, too, since family and friends are so important to us and will be to Ryland as he goes through this transition. He needs to know, without a shadow of a doubt, that he is loved as a boy, just as he was as a girl. If you would like to learn more about gender-nonconforming or transgender children, some recommended books are "The Transgender Child" by Stephanie Brill and Rachel Pepper, and "Gender Born, Gender Made—Raising Healthy Gender-Nonconforming Children" by Dr. Diane Ehrensaft. We have also found the website Gender Spectrum very helpful: http://www.genderspectrum.org/.

Additionally, I highly recommend the documentary, "Trans," which you can borrow from us or purchase at http://www.transthemovie.com/.

We realize this is an incredibly long message, but the topic deserved an in-depth explanation for many reasons, the least of which is that we value and love you, in the same way we want you to value and love Ryland. Honestly, in the grand scheme of things, Ryland's gender variance is just one of many attributes, one that will certainly challenge us, but teach us in ways we can only imagine right now. We are so lucky to have two, healthy and happy kids. Relative to the horrific things that other people have to endure with their children all over the world, this is nothing.

Hillary & Jeff

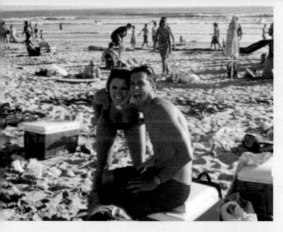

The day that Jeff and I met on the beaches of San Diego. That day made me a believer in love at first sight.

By far the most significant part of our wedding day was having my brother (Ryan) and the rest of the family together for one of the last days of his life.

DMZ Visual Marketing & Photography

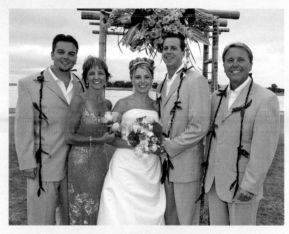

My brother gave the warmest and longest hugs that made you *feel* how much he cared. He later said that my wedding day "was the best day of his life."

DMZ Visual Marketing & Photography

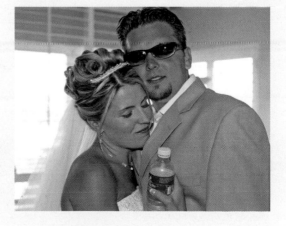

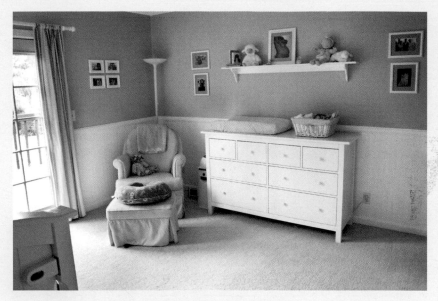

We were so excited when we learned that we were having a little girl, and we immediately went to work on the perfect nursery plan.

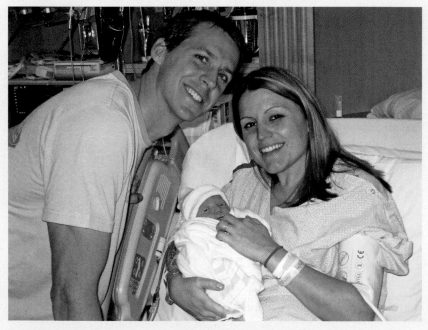

Ryland's arrival was one of the happiest days of my life. Becoming a mother was one of my biggest dreams.

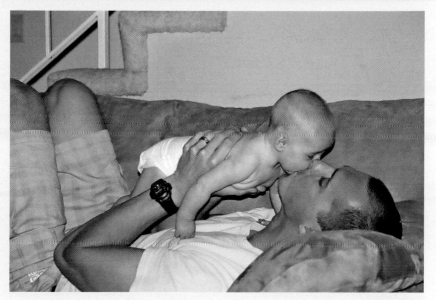

Jeff has always been a very involved, hands-on, and loving father. From the very beginning, he has wanted to be present for every milestone or fall.

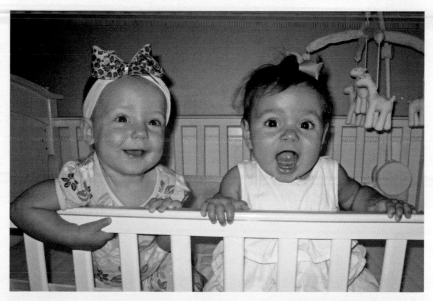

Meeting Jenn and Gianna came at a perfect time. Ryland and Gianna quickly became friends and continue to share an unbreakable bond.

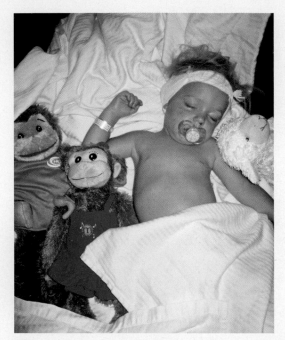

We knew the day of Ryland's cochlear implant surgery would be difficult, but we also knew we made the right choice.

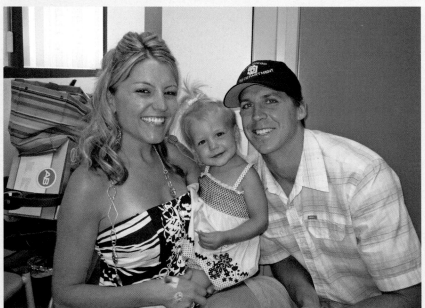

The day Ryland was "turned on" came with much anticipation, and eventually Ryland grew to love the new sensation of hearing.

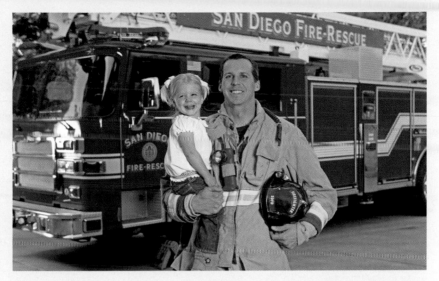

Visiting Jeff at the firehouse was one of Ryland's favorite outings, but our visits became less frequent as Ryland progressed through transition.

Image provided courtesy of Advanced Bionics. Photograph by Gilles Mingasson.

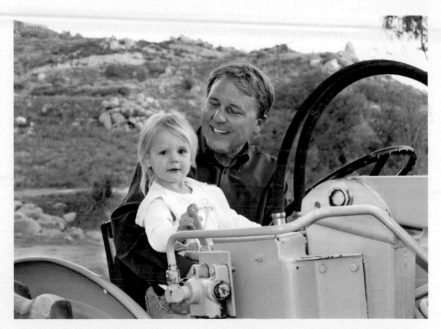

Visiting Grandma and Grandpa on their ranch was always something Ryland looked forward to.

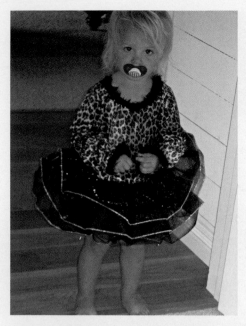

You can see the sadness in Ryland's eyes, at age 2, when we forced her to wear feminine costumes.

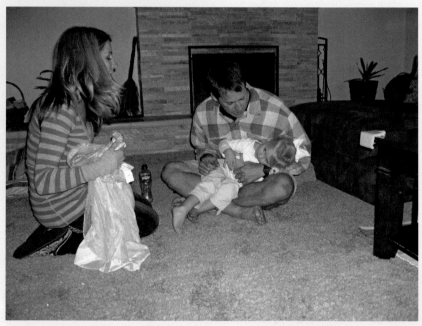

Ryland would try every tactic to avoid wearing dresses, and I would often have to "coach" her for weeks leading up to an event.

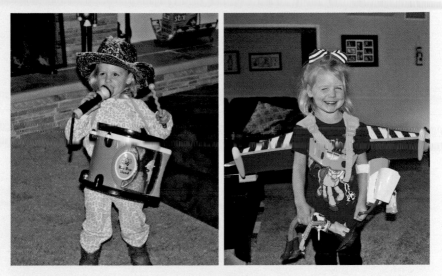

Left: Ryland loved to dress up as a cowboy, not a cowgirl, as often as possible.
Right: Santa provided Ryland with her favorite *Toy Story* Christmas gifts this year.

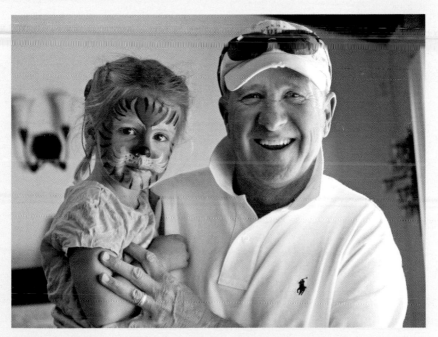

Whenever Ryland was given an option for face painting, she continuously chose superheroes or dangerous animals.

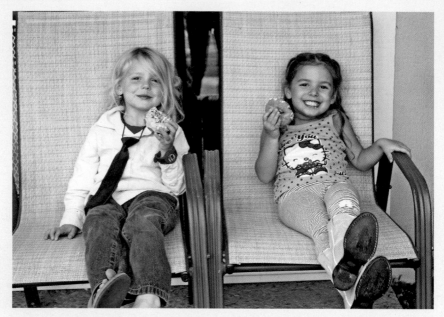

Ryland and Gianna always got along great during playdates.

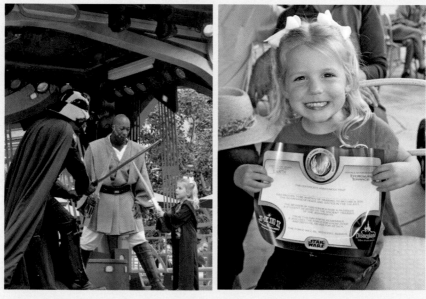

The highlight of Ryland's fifth birthday at Disneyland was when both she and Gianna were chosen to go onstage for the light saber battle with Darth Vader.

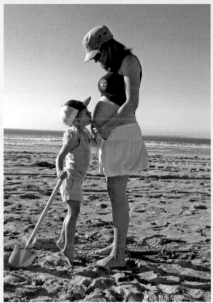

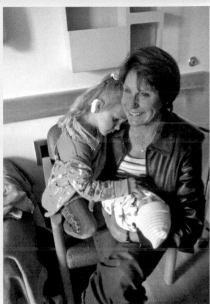

Left: Ryland was so excited to share her life with a little sister.
Right: Ryland and my mother-in-law, Peg, the day after Brynley arrived.

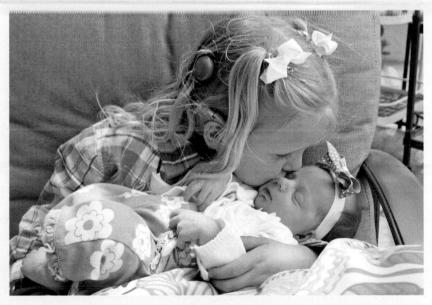

Though we agreed on mostly boy clothes for the day-to-day, there continued to be a struggle on big holidays, like the Easter after Brynley was born.

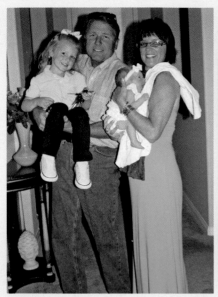

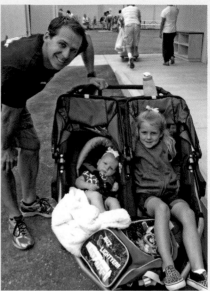

Left: Both Ryland and Brynley's baby showers were canceled due to preterm labor and bed rest, so my mom finally had the chance to shower us *after* Brynley arrived.

Right: Ryland on her first day of transitional kindergarten. She often zipped her sweatshirt up to cover any shirts she didn't like.

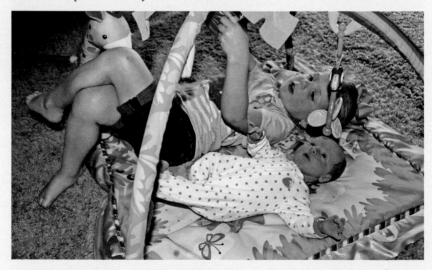

From the moment Brynley arrived home from the hospital, Ryland began talking to her like an equal and coaching her on how to be a good person.

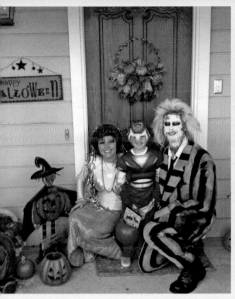
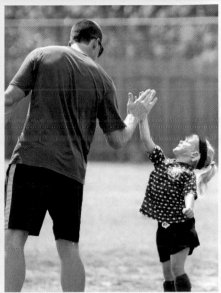

Left: For many transgender kids, Halloween can be their favorite holiday. Ryland chose to be Iron Man, and ended up meeting a boy with the same name and costume.

Right: Jeff went out and bought a matching purple assistant-coach shirt so that Ryland wouldn't feel uncomfortable playing in her uniform.

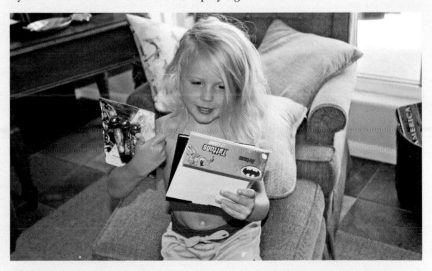

Though Ryland hadn't transitioned yet, most of our friends and family knew of her desire to only play with those items typically considered to be for a boy.

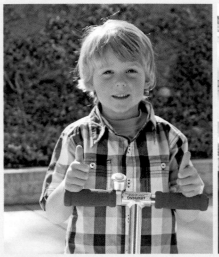

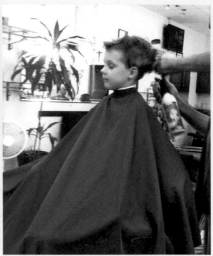

Left: Ryland's very first professional boy haircut brought out an entirely different child.

Right: Ryland was so excited when he was able to get his hair cut at Jeff's barbershop.

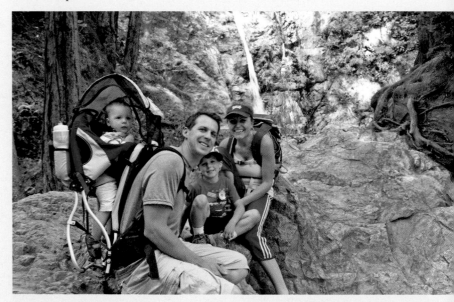

Our first nuclear-family vacation was monumental and pivotal on our journey. The simple tasks of cooking meals together made us remember the pleasures in life and removed us from the chaos of back home.

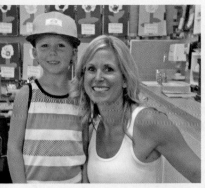
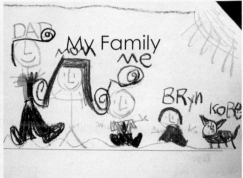

Left: Ryland and his teacher Mrs. Dodds, who was his protector and second Mama Bear when I released him into the gates of school.

Right: From the very beginning, Ryland has always drawn himself as a boy within any self- or family portraits.

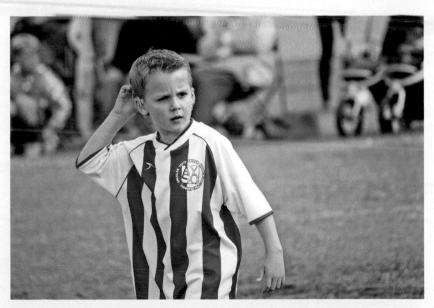

Once Ryland transitioned, we signed him up for the boy's soccer team. He was so much happier playing against some of the boys from his kindergarten class.

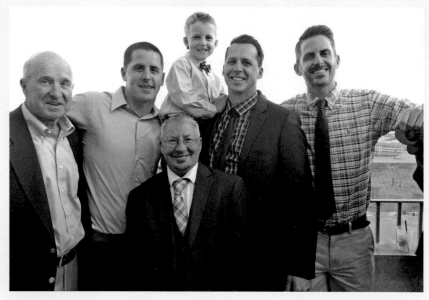

Jeff, Grandpa Rand, Uncle Jay, Uncle Scott, Connor, and Ryland posing for a "guys only" picture at the Nicky Awards in San Diego.

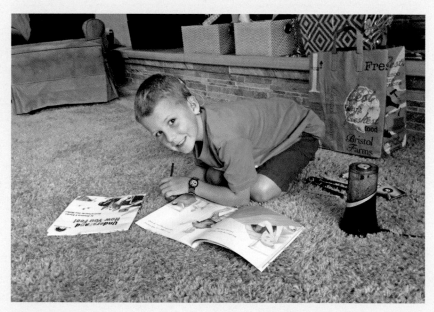

Ryland is coloring a book sent by one of the many kind supporters who have sent emails, letters, and even care packages to our family.

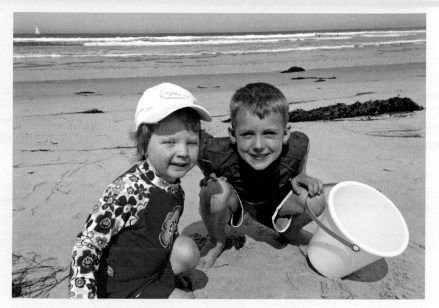

Ryland and his sister posing for a picture on the San Diego sands where it all began.

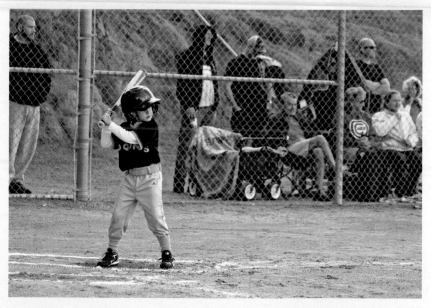

The perfected baseball stance that I love so much. It warms my heart to see him fitting in and playing with all of the other boys in the league.

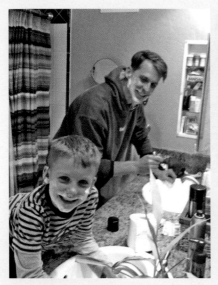

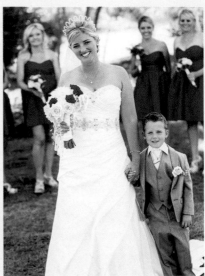

Left: A child shaving kit (no blade, of course) was clearly one of Ryland's favorite gifts for Christmas this year.

Right: Our dearest friend Macie's wedding was incredibly special, as she honored Ryland by asking him to be her ring-bearer. *Kristina Chartier Photography*

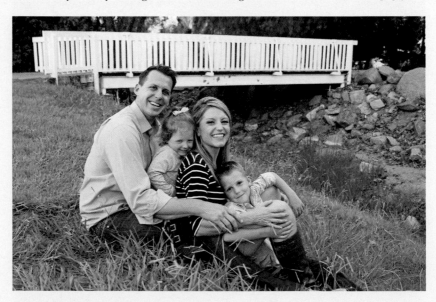

Our joyful family, after navigating down some difficult roads and finding peace through love, understanding, and acceptance. *Vikki Dinh Photography*

Chapter Nine

Shaping the Future

We send the letter out on January 25, 2013, ten days after Ryland's haircut. That same day, we also call Ryland's school and set up an urgent meeting with the principal and staff. The school environment will be one of the most crucial areas for us to try to establish a kind and loving foundation for our child.

We gather in the conference room of Ryland's school. Jeff stands by me as I tearfully tell the school officials that Ryland has gender dysphoria. "What that means," I tell them, "is that Ryland is transgender." Most of them listen with compassion in their faces, while it's clear the principal, Mr. Kane, is processing how it will be necessary for the school to deal with it. I don't give him any room to guess: one of the most pressing tasks, I tell them, is to take down the girl and boy bathroom signs in Ryland's transitional kindergarten classroom. They agree to cover up the bathroom signs in Ryland's class so that he isn't singled out or reprimanded for still using the girls' bathroom even though he's a boy. The kids all know the girls' bathroom from the boys', and in 2013, there are no laws in place to guarantee that Ryland will be able to use the restroom of his choice. Most of his classmates still see him as a little girl—a tomboy— who prefers being with the boys. For now, as far as we can tell, Ryland isn't quite confident enough to begin using the boys' bathroom.

In the meeting, Mrs. Sayers also speaks up and says she will begin referring to Ryland as "Ryland," instead of "he" or "she." "I'll also just say a quick sentence or two to the class to explain that some kids have the brain of the opposite gender," she says, "and that will be that."

I appreciate the support with which Mrs. Sayers is willing to navigate this huge change in a prekindergarten class. She seems to get that she has to be assertive, kind, and yet as low-key as possible when addressing this with the children. Kids are much smarter than we give them credit for. If she were to say nothing, they'd probably just go home with even more questions, and their confusion would lead to confusion among their parents, and all that would just make all this harder for Ryland.

The meeting is very emotional and I let myself break into tears several times throughout, but by the end, Jeff and I are satisfied that the staff have all accepted the situation and agreed to deal with it as appropriately as possible. Before we leave, I give all of them a copy of the letter we wrote, along with Darlene's contact information and a handout that Darlene gave us:

Some people are born with BOY bodies, and have the hearts and brains of GIRLS.

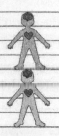

Some people are born with GIRL bodies, and have the hearts and brains of BOYS.

When this happens, the person can feel sad. ☹

It makes them happier to change the way people see them to match how they feel inside their hearts and brains.

People who were born with boy bodies but have the hearts and brains of girls want to be seen as a girl. They want to be called by a girl name. They want other people to say "she" instead of "he" and "her" instead of "him".

People who were born with girl bodies but have the hearts and brains of boys want to be seen as a boy. They want to be called by a boy name. They want other people to say "he" instead of "she" and "him" instead of "her".

When people they love use the names and the words they want, they feel really happy. ☺

Created by Darlene Tando, LCSW
www.DarleneTando.com

I also get permission from Mrs. Sayers and Mr. Kane to hand out the worksheet, stapled to the letter, to the parents and caregivers of the children in Ryland's class.

At home, we begin to change Ryland's bedroom to look more like a little boy's bedroom. He and Brynley will still share a bedroom, but I'm going to have to get a little creative in blending their two styles.

He is beyond excited when we walk into Target to choose a new comforter for his bed. "Mom, look! I want that one right there!" he says, pointing to the top shelf. We agree on a comforter with blue, brown, and green plaid, and we grab stuffed dinosaurs to set on his bed and figurines to decorate his side of the room.

At home, when we place the last dinosaur figure on his shelf, Ryland lies on his bed and glances over to me, wearing a huge smile. His bedroom finally mirrors a room that a brother shares with his little sister, and he's proud and content with his new sleeping quarters. For me, it's a powerful experience that actually feels like a rebirth—we hadn't touched much of the decoration in this room since we were adorning it for our little girl. This new change might actually allow us all to sleep a little more peacefully at night.

With the aesthetics of the room complete, I go through his drawers, stacking all the girls' clothes into a plastic storage bin for Brynley to wear one day. Maybe all the pink and ruffles will find some use in the next couple of years.

We do all we can think of to begin to give Ryland the confidence that he's now seen as a little boy. Not everything about the transition goes smoothly, though. I'm getting very little sleep, maybe three or four hours a night, as I feed Brynley and then lie awake pondering the mixed responses we're getting from people who received our letter.

Many are outstanding—both sides of our family are now completely on board, and a few of our neighbors and some of the parents of kids in Ryland's class have written back to us and said that their kids love playing with Ryland, and they just want to clarify whether they should be using male pronouns now. We always thank them, and answer yes to this question. The mom of Ryland's kindergarten "boyfriend" emails me to say that she's trying to explain to her son that Ryland can't be his girlfriend anymore, but Ryland can be his best friend now. "Brandon still wants to marry his best friend," she says. "I thinks that's so sweet, and we can just work on that later." She asks me out for lunch so that we can really explain to our boys what this means for their friendship now. Another mom even tells me that she has a close friend who is very well known in the San Diego transgender community, if we ever need additional support.

But some of the responses are very hurtful, with moms asking things like, "What if Ryland changes her mind when she's older and wants to go back to being a girl?" One mom in our neighborhood has sipped wine with me while her son, who's allergic to peanuts, had a playdate with Ryland in our home. When discussing her son's allergy, she'd told me, "I wrote a letter to his teacher and requested that none of the children bring anything with nuts in their lunches—peanut butter, trail mix, nuts themselves— nothing. The school has to comply, and if anybody doesn't like it, then who cares what they think?" she said.

But after she hears about our letter regarding Ryland, at the park she flips her hair at me and says, "I don't really get why you decided to bring a personal issue into your child's school." *Isn't the well-being of our children personal to us?* I want to ask her. *Isn't that why there's a school-wide nut ban where your son goes?!* Instead, I'm so dumbfounded by her nerve that I say nothing.

Others cite their interpretations of what the Bible says about sexuality—one mom invites me to lunch at Subway near the kids' school, and then corners me when we're seated in a booth with our sandwiches. "I suppose you're wondering why I invited you here," she says.

Uncomfortable, and trying to adjust to all this new vulnerability that our letter has brought on, I tell her, "Yes, I guess I am."

"I have never known anyone gay or lesbian," she says, "and I don't know how you have raised your children . . . but my husband and I have raised our children to believe in the Lord."

Oh boy.

"God created Adam and Eve—a man and a woman. Elizabeth came home from school yesterday and told me that Ryland is a boy now. I explained to Elizabeth that this is not possible—because God created men and women."

I begin to break down inside, fighting my hardest to hold in the tears. This woman has taken advantage of this opportunity to rip me apart because she's afraid of what it means if life is not black-and-white, if to be a man or a woman is more complicated than the parts that God gives us. *This is the world we live in,* I tell myself. People are afraid to talk to their children, sometimes for fear they will put this "transgender thing" in their child's head and that the child will "catch it." A child is only transgender if they are insistent, persistent, and consistent when they express their gender as being incongruent with their body parts. Many people, like Caitlyn Jenner, transition much later in life, and when this is the case, they almost always say that they knew since the time they were a child that they were the opposite gender on the inside. No transgender person has the same experience as another. And no parent of a transgender kid, or any kid, has my experience.

I put down my sandwich and make a decision: I will not let anyone push me around, using God or anything as their excuse to judge my son or our family.

"Funny you mention God," I tell her. "I have spent my entire life being taught something similar, going to church, believing in the Bible. But tell me this: what would you do if your child said to you, 'Why did God make me like this?'"

She sits, silently, no expression on her face.

I continue: "This has been an awful thing to go through, I assure you, and I don't have all of the answers, but I do know that I have exhausted all the resources. This is my only option to save my child's life and honestly, I never thought I would be in this position, but here I am. I am going to make the best of it. *You* tell *me* what I should do?!"

Still, silence.

The defense rests.

I leave my sandwich and walk out. We have been through so much, and now my morals are being called into question? The family values that Jeff and I have are stronger than some families: *We will love our children no matter what.*

I know that I haven't convinced this woman that I'm not crazy, but at least she got a little piece of my stressful life. She has no idea that she—as a Christian—is causing my life—as a Christian—to be much more difficult than it needs to be. *"Jesus loves everyone!"* I want to scream. *"And God doesn't make mistakes!"*

Every morning for the next few weeks on my drive taking

Ryland to school, I have to pull off to the side of the road to get sick. Each day, I panic that I'll run into her again. It's inevitable, but when the time comes, I hope there are enough other moms close by who will keep me engaged enough not to have to address her.

After a few weeks, my cousin Melissa texts me. I hadn't heard much from her after her response to our letter when all she replied was something along the lines of how Jeff and I have a tough road ahead, no matter which path we choose. I knew she was struggling with the change; she'd been raised even more conservatively than I was and she's concerned about Ryland's future, but her response was far less than I'd hoped for, given how close and unconditional our relationship has always been. With so much support and praise pouring in from all around us, it broke my heart to feel like I didn't have the full support from someone whom I considered to be a sister. I knew that I needed to give her space, and I'm so happy when I see my phone displaying a text message from her. However, as I open the text, my heart sinks. My sadness turns to anger when I read what she's stating: she would like to make Brynley the flower-girl in her wedding instead of Ryland. Then she signs off with an *LOL*.

LOL? Whoa. Is that her attempt to keep this light? Trying to give her the chance to express her perspective, I reply, "What about Ryland?"

She responds by telling me that she already has a ring bearer, and she intends to keep things the way they are.

I'm dumbfounded. Angry. I know that Andrew comes from a family that has devout Christian morals, and I certainly know what it's like to marry into a big, strong, loving family. Maybe she wants to avoid an uncomfortable situation at her wedding. Maybe this is even her way of trying to help Ryland. Still, that doesn't make it any easier for me to accept that Ryland will no longer be a part of the most important day of her life. Ryland will be so crushed if I say, "Hey, Aunt Melissa is replacing you in the wedding because you are transitioning to a boy and she has no place for you anymore." I'm not willing to tell Ryland that this is going on, for fear it will dim his shining new light. I'm so angry that anyone dare hurt him, especially Melissa. Out of frustration with texting about such a sensitive and serious matter, I pick up the phone and dial her. Immediately, I lose any ounce of composure I've been maintaining. I begin screaming and yelling, and with every word that flies from my mouth is the knowledge that I will regret this later. We hang up the phone, and I send her one final text: "I hope your wedding day goes well, but we will not be attending." My heart sinks as I press SEND, but I feel as though I have no other choice. I have to protect my child and his feelings.

This text will be the last mutual exchange of communication between Melissa and me for years to come.

IN THE MIDDLE of all these big changes, Ryland gets a ruptured eardrum and runs a massive fever. I can't help but wonder if this is his body's way of manifesting the stress he's experiencing under the surface during this transition in front of everyone he knows. We find a new pediatrician, an amazing woman, who promptly prescribes antibiotic drops. I know she's the doctor I've been longing for when she immediately agrees to write an official doctor's letter that states that Ryland is transgender. Her son has a friend in his eighth-grade class who's a transgender girl. "My son thinks it's no big deal!" she says. "The kids are all okay with it."

During this time, I feel as if we're in survival mode—there's so much coming at us that in an effort to keep from lashing out at Jeff in pain every time I sense judgment from someone, he and I begin to simply coexist and operate like business partners. We're sticking together, and we never stop loving each other, but as individuals, we're both going through so much turmoil that it's difficult for both of us to think of the other person. I feel like I have a teammate, but I'm still so hurt that I know if I lean on him too heavily and he lets me down, it will be very hard on our relationship. Because he's so often at work, it's me who's forced to deal with the day-to-day reactions we're receiving, and Jeff relies on what I'm able to relay to him. However, he and I are deeply appreciative when the people with whom we surround ourselves reach out to tell us that they support us. The help we need always arrives just at the moment we need it most.

To add to all the pressure, we're invited to speak to the audiology students at the University of California, San Diego (UCSD) about Ryland's experience with cochlear implants. I prepare my talk carefully for the students, trying to figure out how we can show video of Ryland's progress with hearing and speech unless we explain why the footage from the beginning of Ryland's life shows him as a little girl. Since his deaf diagnosis at age one, we've compiled multiple videos that document Ryland's journey, and we've always been willing to share this with other families of deaf children and experts who work in a field related to audiology. But now, for the first time, we're faced with an unusual challenge.

"Hillary . . . you know we need to show these videos," Jeff says, "but if we go in there and try to revert back to *she* for this entire presentation, it isn't going to work." I know he's right. "You know what's going to happen," he says. "We're going to slip up and use *he*. It's going to make things very awkward for the audience, and besides . . . it doesn't feel right to go back."

"I agree. What do you think?"

"I think we have to address it. I think we have to tell them why we are going to be referring to Ryland as *he*. I thing we need to put it all out there, regardless of the reactions we may get."

I know that it's going to open the door to a lot of questions, but I know he's right. It needs to be done.

We rework our speech, and as we stand before the students that day, we are extremely nervous. After the "thank you for having us here" opening, Jeff states to the class: "There is one thing that we've decided that we need to address and put out there, or we are going to add a lot of confusion to this speech," he says. The class looks at him with some concern in their faces. My husband continues. "Over the course of the last couple years, we have been through a lot more with Ryland than just his deaf diagnosis. We have also discovered that Ryland is also transgender."

My heart races. This is the first time we've ever opened up and come out in front of a large audience. As Jeff speaks, I scan the room for reactions. Surprisingly, we haven't lost them yet.

"You may find it odd that we are bringing this up," he continues, "but because it is such a new transition for our family, you may hear us inadvertently and purposefully move between the *he* and *she* pronouns. We knew that if we didn't say something to explain all this to you, we would cause some confusion. We want to make sure we stay on the topic today, but if any of you have questions on this part of our journey, we'd be more than happy to answer any questions at the end."

There's a brief moment of silence and we quickly see an understanding and appreciation move over the audience. A few squirm in their seats, but I know for the most part, we are understood. It's relieving, and empowering. For the first time, we have stood together and made our situation known. We know that we're offering a gift to these students by presenting our personal struggles and accomplishments on Ryland's hearing journey. We never realized we would also be receiving a "gift" from a student in the class that would further strengthen our ability to tell our story.

Dear Mr. and Mrs. Whittington,

My name's Charles, and I'm one of the audiology students you shared your story about Ryland with yesterday. I just wanted to thank you again for the presentation, and thank you for being such compassionate, level-headed people and parents. As well as gaining a new insight into the world of hearing parents with a deaf child, I also got a glimpse into the process of learning to understand and accept a trans child. I have several friends in the trans community, and hearing about the prejudice, injustice, and hate they face on a nearly daily basis is heartbreaking. That's just one reason your story was so moving.

I know it wasn't easy to educate yourselves, understand, and eventually accept Ryland's identity. I'm so proud of you. You've given me hope that these times of ignorance and misunderstanding may one day come to a close, thanks to loving and forward-thinking parents like yourselves. Your actions give the entire queer community hope that someday they won't have to fear abandonment by their loved ones and guardians, and that someday acceptance will be commonplace. As the parents of this generation, you are shaping the future: a future where love is paramount and queer youth can feel like they belong. So again, thank you. You're not just parents. You're heroes.

All my best,
Charles

In my response to Charles, I tell him:

I have never been called a "hero" and never been told by someone I just met that they were proud of me. So thank you! It's amazing what a few weeks of transition has done for my son, my marriage, my hope, and my strength to keep going and fighting for these kids. I appreciate your kind words, and your interest in our crazy life!

I think it's fun to be different, and I hope that we can keep in touch.

Warmest,
Hillary

This letter that we receive after we give our talk is completely unexpected . . . and it's my first piece of evidence that we can actually help improve someone's life by sharing Ryland's story. For a moment, I don't feel lonely. I feel honored.

Chapter Ten

Gender Spectrum

By early February, my skin has grown a little thicker, and the uplifting words continue to pour in. Ryland's speech therapist, Gwen—who has a young person in her life who is gay—writes us to say, "I know this was so incredibly difficult for you and that you both want the best for Ryland. Your family is in my prayers."

Matt and Michelle write to say, "Let's get our boys together soon!"

Aunt Sue says, "Hillary and Jeff, what wonderful parents you are! There is nothing harder than not to be true to who you really are. Let me know what I can do to help. I can't wait to play boy games and climb trees together. Love to all of you!"

Even my uncle, who's Mormon, writes, "We are all God's children made in his image and we'll love Ryland for who he is unconditionally."

We send out a follow-up letter thanking our loved ones for their support:

We are so touched by the support from everyone. It is such
a relief to have it all out there, and we are feeling loved.
Though we didn't hear from everyone, we still understand
it takes processing time. We understand it will be difficult
getting used to "he/him" pronouns and Ryland is very un-
derstanding. We think he appreciates the effort more than
anything. We love you and hope to see you very soon!

By all accounts, Ryland's transition at school is going as
smoothly as we could have prayed. Some of the children, in
their brilliant innocence, have taken immediately to embracing
Ryland as a boy. From what we can tell, it seems that most of the
others just continue to think of Ryland the way they always did:
as a friend. The children have amazed us with their instant acceptance. It seems that to them, a kid's a kid—just another playmate to have fun with.

At home, there are adjustments that we continue to make, as
we're quickly learning that there's an endless stream of to-dos for
parents who have accommodated their child in making a transition and affirming their gender identity. We're attending to legal-
related matters, like deciding whether we need to change the
gender on Ryland's birth certificate—for now, we don't. When I
research it, I find that it will take quite a lot of legal effort, and it's
just a step that emotionally I'm not quite ready to take. Jeff and
I pledge that we'll deal with the birth certificate change once we
get through some of the more pressing emotional, medical, and
legal matters that need to be addressed immediately. We're also
very fortunate to have chosen a gender-neutral name, which has
enabled us to avoid some of the horror stories I've heard at our
support group meetings, like children's birth names being called

out at the doctor or in the classroom. I decide to put off having everything changed legally, including Ryland's middle name.

Sometimes I feel like I have so many issues to deal with that the ones causing me the least grief in any given moment are pushed to the bottom of the list.

Though we're facing a lot of new hurdles with Ryland's transition, his speech has progressed to the point that we're able to cut back on his speech therapy appointments. It's a much-needed and welcomed relief.

A national group leader at TransYouth Family Allies has advised us to create what she calls a "safe folder." This is a portfolio that parents compile to document proof that a child is truly transgender, should Child Protection Services ever be called to intervene. For us it would be proof that Jeff and I are not forcing our child to live a life of gender nonconformity against his will. In the folder, we would include letters from our new pediatrician, as well as Darlene Tando, the leaders of the Transforming Family support group, and other close family and friends. We are also advised to include self-portraits in which Ryland has depicted himself as a boy, snapshots of him from over the years presenting as a boy, and background checks on Jeff and me from the state Justice Department to demonstrate that we're not criminally deviant. Truthfully, I only get so far in completing the folder, out of frustration that it even needs to be created. We find a level of absurdity to have to provide so much evidence of our child's identity. I feel as though our parenting is in question, when a five-minute visit with our child would be enough to prove to anyone that he's happy, healthy, and well-adjusted.

Then there are the more practical aspects of life with a child who is newly transitioned. Right after we cut Ryland's hair, he asked that I remove any reminiscence of his past from around the home. I went around and took down all of the photos that featured him as a girl, but when I saw how blank our walls were, I decided to leave a very select few where he's not shown with a dress on, or bows in his hair. There are also certain family members whom I want to display in photos with Ryland, but I don't want to make Ry uncomfortable. I scour our photo albums and computer files for images of Ryland wearing plain outfits. I use a photography filter app to make them black-and-white, and Ryland is satisfied with the transformations.

I keep some of my old pictures of Ryland and hide them away inside a box in a cupboard . . . and part of me feels like a traitor for doing so. But Jeff and I don't want to destroy every single image of the memories that we all made in the first five years of his life. Ryland is Ryland, and inside he's been the same child at every single phase since his birth. The thought strikes me: inside the home of a family, usually it's the display of photos that shows a child's transformation over time, but in our family, it's the absence of photos that demonstrates Ryland's transformation.

Our taking away the old pictures that portrayed Ryland as female proves to be very significant for Ry. It shows him that we're willing to erase some of the past to make him feel affirmed in the present and accepted as a boy. I don't ever want him to think I miss the prior version of him; he might mistake that for my wish that he were actually a girl.

Yet, the fact is, I can't deny that I will always cherish those early years with my child. I want to remember my baby. I just know that I'm lucky there are only five years of photos to "hide" from Ryland. Some of the families we've met have more time that they have to erase and "unremember." I think this is why some families feel like there is a death when their child transitions. You have to erase the old version you knew so well, and redirect your mind to think of them as a different person altogether. The truth is, that person is still the exact same on the inside. There is no death at all. It's just a new "outer shell" to get used to seeing. With every change this transition calls us to make, we're just glad we're getting used to seeing this sooner rather than later in Ryland's life, and in the life of our family.

But then, of course, there's the challenge of social media. When I begin to post more photos of my kids on Facebook, we receive some interesting comments. Immediately I realize that there are a lot of people who are on my Facebook who are not close enough to us to have received the letter. I go onto Facebook less—not so much because the judgment of others scares me, but because I don't really care to share our private life with people whom I don't trust deep down.

When we're out and about—say, at dinner, grocery shopping, or at the park—acquaintances who heard about the letter approach Jeff and me and applaud our unconditional love for our child. One common theme they express to us is that they don't know how to explain Ryland's transition to their children, and many of them come to us for help. I often refer them to the diagram that Darlene gave us, and I wish we had the time to meet individually with every single person during this time.

Some people have had the nerve to approach us and ask if or when Ryland will get a sex change, and each time, my stomach has dropped. We find it completely absurd that people have the nerve or audacity to inquire about our child's genitalia. Frankly, it's none of their business, and it feels as awkward as if we were to ask them about *their* child's private parts. Though we understand the curiosity, we don't feel these questions deserve a response. Jeff and I have discussed this at great length and when it comes to this sort of procedure, the answer is simple: we're talking about Ryland's body, and if and when the time comes to make that decision, then it's completely up to him.

I put up a strong façade to protect everyone—including myself—but truthfully, I'm still trying not to crumble to the ground. I'm overwhelmed, stressed out, and going through my own form of grieving. I never feel relief from my worries that Ryland will be bullied or left out for being transgender, and the books I've read have validated my feeling that while I've certainly gained a happy, healthy son, I've lost my former little girl. I've buried my own visions for his future and I need time, probably a *lot* of time, to grow used to the fact that Ryland may never have children, as I'd imagined that my daughter would. I'd always imagined him having biological children, and I'm surprised at how very caught up I am on this detail in the transition. Part of the challenge of letting Ryland transition so young is that I don't think he understands that he will most likely never be able to procreate biologically. One of my most meaningful roles in life is my role as a mother. A fear throbs inside me that Ryland won't get to experience this same sense of accomplishment if he realizes one day that he wants to have children.

Knowing that I can't break down crying in front of the kids, I take to long jogs or car rides alone. I also let the tears flow whenever I'm in the shower. I do not want anyone to know how much this entire process hurts me. It is testing my deepest strength and endurance in life.

"RYLAND, HURRY UP and get your cleats and mitt!" I yell from the kitchen. "We're going to be late for your first day of baseball!"

Baseball is the sport that Ryland has wanted to play more than all the others, and in the spring after his transition, he's finally getting his chance. At registration, we requested that he would be placed in the tee-ball league since it was his first year playing, but at his first practice, we immediately realized we'd made a big mistake. Ryland was a full head taller, faster, and more mature than the four- and five-year-olds on his team. He's six, but emotionally, he's even beyond his years. It would have been a disservice for us to hold him back with kids so little. To see his friends and classmates all playing baseball in the Rookie League together would have devastated him. After that first week, we asked if he could be moved back up to the correct league for his age group.

That's Ryland: every time we fear that he's not quite ready for a new stage, he proves us wrong by a mile. When his first base-ball practice rolls around, I quickly gather water, snacks, and Brynley's baby doll and stroller, and we all rush out the door. I hate for us to be late to anything, especially when we're still in first-impression mode.

We're actually on time when I pull up to the little baseball field, nestled in the middle of the beautiful neighborhood of Mount Helix. It almost looks like a scene from an old Ameri-can movie when you round the corner of Russell Road and drive down to the field. The trees surrounding the little field are mature and beautiful.

Ryland jogs to the dugout, where I stand by just long enough to make sure the coach is acquainted with him. On the bleach-ers, I position myself so I can watch Brynley and keep my eye on Ryland at the same time.

Practice begins. Brynley scales up and down the bleachers,

runs around with the other little girls, and hangs on my legs, smiling up at me for attention.

It suits me to keep my socializing to my little girl . . . I'm not in my usual social mood today. When I make eye contact with the other moms, I smile cordially, but I don't feel like putting myself in a position to share my feelings or Ryland's story.

About twenty minutes into practice, I see a cute little guy running toward the dugout to join in. The coach looks at his watch, as if the child has any control over his mom's errands schedule. He's tall for his age, with short blond hair and dark-rimmed glasses. The coach points him toward the field and the little boy smiles, taking a position not too far from Ryland.

A tall, thin, blond woman walks toward me and sits down right next to me. She's pretty—very little makeup, light freckles on her face, pearly white teeth. Normally, I would immediately strike up a conversation and become friends . . . but not today.

Another mom walks up and takes a seat on my other side. The two women strike up a conversation. I try to keep to myself, even though I'm physically positioned directly between the two of them.

Then I see Ryland running toward me out of left field. Either he has to use the bathroom or the battery on his cochlear implant has died. With his baseball mitt tucked under his arm, he whispers in my ear. "Mom, I have to pee." The look on his face is worried.

His coach runs over to the bleachers. "I don't think I have a key to the bathrooms here. Does he have to pee or . . ." He makes a face as if to say, *Does he have to go number two?*

"I have to pee," Ryland says.

"Well, you're a boy," the coach chuckles. "Go use the bushes over there!"

Inside, my anxiety spikes. *Bushes over where?* We're standing in the middle of a quaint little neighborhood and I have seconds before my child pees his pants. What am I going to do with no public restroom and a little boy who can't stand up to urinate like the rest of the little boys here?!

Instantly, I grab Ryland's hand and pretend to walk toward the bushes that border between the parking lot and the field. Instead, I hurry to the back of my SUV and inside the hatch, I set up my mini potty chair that I have carried around since Ry was a toddler. I quickly line the potty chair with the disposable plastic bag and close the hatch of my trunk as fast as possible so no one sees what we're doing or where we are.

Brynley! I left Brynley over there in my mad dash to the car!

I race around the side of my car to locate my little girl. If she can't find me and has a meltdown, Ryland will be busted with his pants down and we'll all be in big trouble!

Okay—there she is, playing with another little girl not far from the bushes. I peek into my trunk to see Ryland's progress. He's ducking down, trying to get his baseball belt and pants up without anyone seeing him. I open the back and slide my body inside.

"Mom, stop! I'm not done yet!"

"I know—I'm going to help you." Quickly, I help Ry buckle his baseball pants and fasten his black belt inside the loops of his baseball pants. He hops out of the back and runs back onto the field.

I sit back down on the bleachers. The cute mom to my left says with a big smile, "Don't you just love having boys so they can go in the bushes?!"

I feel my face go flush. With an uncomfortable laugh I reply, "Yeah, I sure do."

Immediately I rise and go to swoop up Brynley—the most convincing way to change the subject. I'm just relieved that I pulled it all off without anyone sensing that something is up with us, but I'm not sure how much longer I can. It feels as though I cannot emotionally deal with explaining our situation one more time.

Shortly after the transition, Jeff's parents purchase the first-ever waterproof cochlear implants so that Ryland can take swim lessons with sound for the first time in his life. Ryland is resistant, and while we try to understand why, I drop off a letter at his swim school out of anticipation that he'll return to his lessons sometime soon.

I get no response, which doesn't shock me, per se, because the owners of the swim school are a quiet, religious family. We were thankful when they were so willing to teach Ryland to swim using hand cues and some sign language.

Maybe they just never opened the letter, I think to myself. But . . . it's kind of a big deal that they understand Ryland has to be addressed as "he" when he begins his lessons again.

One day when I'm chatting with another mom during one of Brynley's "tadpole" toddler lessons, the wife from the family who owns the swim school approaches me. "I haven't seen Ryland in a while," she says. "How's she doing?"

It means a lot that she wants to know about Ryland, but I feel myself drop into a mini panic attack. Has she not read the letter? Did she miss it somehow? Do I need to take her aside?

"He is doing great," I tell her nonchalantly, worried that the mom I've been chatting with will wonder why the instructor has just referred to Brynley's big brother as *she*. Quickly I change the subject. "How have you and your family been?"

Run-ins like this prompt me to begin to carry copies of our

letter in my purse so if I run into someone who doesn't know about the transition, I can hand it to them and invite them to read it when they have time. At Chuck E. Cheese, we run into a mom from Ryland's earliest swimming lessons. She asks me: "Where's Ryland? Who is *that*?" I reach into my purse and hand her the letter. "Great to see you!" I tell her, and Ryland and I scuttle out to the car, where Jeff is buckling Brynley into her car seat.

I've learned not to try to explain this to an acquaintance in person. It's awful for both parties when someone doesn't know what in the world to say, and I end up feeling like I'm on trial. There are times when I have to excuse myself to go hyperventilate, or I break into a sweat with a panic attack when I run into someone and try to remember whether they've gotten the memo. I begin to realize that maybe the letter wasn't quite enough—for Ryland's sake, I have to stop "scuttling" in hurried shame. I have to start walking the walk. I have to "come out" to everyone we know. As Lori Duron wrote in *Raising My Rainbow,* the person with a secret gives up their burden once the secret is out. If we come clean, maybe I can breathe.

Literally.

My mission becomes less about whether any given person supports us and more about showing Ryland that we're standing with him. He's watching every time I encounter someone who doesn't recognize him, who wasn't close enough to be on our email list. Instead of worrying so much about their reactions, I make polite conversation and smile as I give them the envelope. "Here," I tell them. "Read this and get back to me when you can."

BY NOW, BRYNLEY is impossible to keep up with, and in June 2013 Kobe has gotten ill. Our vet helps us determine that he needs to be put down, and Jeff, Ryland, and I are all devastated. "Is there anything more we could possibly pile onto our plate right now?" Jeff says, taking a break from digging a grave for Kobe in our yard while Ryland assists him. "This is turning into Hellville."

I can't disagree with him—things are really rough. As usual, we receive help right when it feels like the balance in our lives might give out completely. Through our LGBT resources, we find out that in July 2013, there's a Gender Spectrum Conference near San Francisco. The mission of the conference is to offer resources and insights to gender-nonconforming youth and their families. Jeff and I eagerly register and book a flight for him, Ryland, and me to go while Brynley stays with Peg and Rand. Jeff signs up for a dads-only breakout session ("very raw," he says later; "Some dads were opening up for the first time, and crying . . . it was really tough") and a workshop that covers the top ten fears among parents of gender-nonconforming children. I sign up for a workshop on writing to deal with fear and a session on surgical options. Together we attend a medical panel, a session on how to maximize support within the school system, and a lecture called "Gender & Faith."

The experience is unreal. There are tons of other kids and parents—new friends for Ryland and a new network of support for Jeff and me. I take note that most of the kids who are around Ryland's age are transgender girls (meaning they were assigned male at birth because of their body parts, and then later transitioned to living in their female gender identity). As one of the expert speakers and I are chatting during a break, I ask her why there are so many more transgender girls than boys. She makes a good point: society is less accepting of gender nonconforming natal males, so parents may discover their child is transgender younger due to being forced to face society's judgments earlier and in a harsher way than Ryland or other undiscovered "tom-boys." Trans girls are often criticized for being little boys who want to wear dresses to school, whereas it's easier for trans boys to slip under the radar as tomboys, that is, until puberty hits and their female body parts begin to develop. This often causes a trans boy to get depressed, angry, and suicidal.

Understanding this makes me feel extremely lucky that we've looked deeper into Ryland's identity than labeling him as a tomboy and ignoring his dysphoria. It also makes me appreciate that Ryland adapted considerably easily to life as a boy. From what the panelists seem to say, a big reason for this is that Jeff and I embraced him that way.

I experience so many emotions on this trip. One of the psy-chologists encourages me to write down one positive thing I do every single day, so I that I can begin to give myself more credit for being a good mom. He encourages me to realize how hard I've been on myself for not allowing Ryland to transition sooner, but there's just nothing that we can do to change that now. I re-member a saying that I recently heard and found very enlighten-ing: "What you allow to control your mind, will." I realize that I need to start honoring my own efforts and accomplishments as a mom more, and I need to do a better job of living in the present. I spend so much time worrying about the future for Ryland—what it will be, what does it mean. Right now, there's nothing I can do about the problems that he may face down the road. We have to take this journey one day at a time and do the best we can for Ryland, Brynley, Jeff, and me every day.

At one of the sessions, we also meet a transgender girl named Devon, whom Ryland recently watched on an episode of Katie Couric's talk show. Devon is a celebrity to Ryland—when he meets her, his face turns red! I can tell that he cannot wait to hug her. When she speaks to him, he's mesmerized by her beauty and confidence. Devon's mom introduces herself to Jeff and me, and as we chat, we discover a surprising connection: her brother-in-law is a firefighter in San Diego who used to be one of Jeff's paramedic instructors and a captain whom he'd worked for on many occasions. Devon's mom gives us her contact information, and we all vow to stay in touch with each other.

By the end of the conference, Jeff and I decide that we'd like to bring the Gender Spectrum founder, Joel Baum, to San Diego to train the staff at Ryland's school. By the time we exit to make our way home, dozens of parents have asked us to provide them with our letter so that they can send it to the people in their children's lives, as well.

On Sunday evening as we fly south toward home, I rest my head back against my seat. I feel completely exhausted and emotionally drained, yet a weight has lifted from me, and I feel something new. It's a sense of authority. A sense of empowerment. For the first time, a strong sense of certainty that we are doing the right thing for our child. Seeing so many other parents with similar stories, fears, and questions made me realize we aren't alone. We actually have more answers and more knowledge than we thought. Ryland was the youngest transgender boy in attendance, and I begin to realize we're pretty seamless and lucky in our journey. Some parents had some pretty awful stories of bullying, self-hate, and suicide attempts. So far, Ryland hasn't experienced anything traumatic.

Maybe we *are* doing something right. Maybe we're not just a family who's *different*. Maybe we're a family who could help change our world.

Chapter Eleven

Heat in the Marriage

We needed that experience leading up to Ryland's start in kindergarten, but I'm caught off guard at kindergarten registration day when a mom whose son will be in Ryland's school stops me in the parking lot. She's petite and soft-spoken—I've seen her in our neighborhood before, and we've shared hellos and a handful of brief conversations. Today, though, it's clear she has an intention. "Hillary?" she says.

I duck my head out of the backseat where I'm buckling Brynley into her car seat. "Oh, hi!"

"Hi," she says. "Hillary, a few months ago, I heard about your letter." *Oh boy,* I think to myself, knowing people have been talking. She goes on. "I need to talk to you."

I brace myself for another lecture on religion or parenting techniques, but instead, she goes on. "I have an older son, named Jackson, who is—well, he's just like Ryland." I feel myself soften in empathy. "He's been hiding in shame for years, wanting to try on my wedding dress, painting his toenails and wearing shoes so his brothers don't see him. He is constantly bullied and made fun of and shows all signs that he's, well, that he's like Ryland. But my husband won't allow it. I don't know what to do."

We stand there talking for a few minutes and make a playdate for our kids so that we can discuss more, and we quickly develop a very trusting friendship. Her middle child, Jackson, accompanies her, and I give him an old pair of my girls' flip-flops. He puts them on immediately. I can tell his mother is conflicted.

Shortly thereafter, it's as though this woman has fallen off the face of the earth. It's clear she's decided to pull back from our friendship as she's battling to keep her family together. In the weeks to follow, I see her and Jackson around the neighborhood, and every time he sees me, he lights up. He knows that Ryland is lucky, and that he will have to hide his feelings—his identity—from his parents and peers. I wish I could adopt him and help him, but getting involved in a family's struggles is playing with fire.

If anyone knows that, it's us. At this stage in Ryland's journey, Jeff and I remain very much on the same page, but that doesn't mean things are smooth. For Jeff, there's still one major aspect of all this that's left jabbing at him: his work.

For the past seven years, Jeff has experienced a *lot* of reward in his profession as a firefighter/paramedic. I can always see it in him—he loves the thrill of the job and the honor it is to be one of the people who are called on to assist someone on what may be the worst day of his or her life. Over the years, Jeff has probably seen more death and destruction than most people will ever see, and he's collected a lot of painful memories and images that we don't care to relive. Unfortunately, he says, it's hard to ever shake these and I'm not sure that he—or I—ever will.

I know the part of his work that he has loved the most is

his bond with his colleagues. In the horrendous experiences and moments you witness and live through together as a firefighter, you tend to build bonds with the people who are by your side—they call each other brothers and sisters. The fire department is their home away from home, and they spend twenty-four hours at a time together . . . sometimes way more. They cook together, eat together, laugh together, relive the pain together, and confide in each other. For a long time, Jeff has considered his crew to be as close to him as our family: they're there to protect and support you, both professionally and personally.

When Ryland arrived nearly one year after Jeff worked his first shift, he started to see the raw reality of things, especially when we found out that Ry was deaf. He came home from work one morning after a large structure fire the night before. "Here I was," he said, "pressed to the floor of this home by the heat of the smoke and fire. I couldn't even see my hand in front of my face." His partner, on the nozzle of the hose line, was inching his way toward the seat of the fire. The chain saws roared above them as the truck crew attempted to cut a hole in the roof to get them some relief from the heat. "Hill," he said, "it hit me: If I die in this fire, I'm leaving a child behind!" From that point, for him, it had to be a job. He began skipping a lot of off-duty get-togethers with the guys, and when he came home, I know that he left as much of what he experienced at the station as he possibly could. Still, it was often very traumatic.

Ryland was still living as a girl back then. He was well known and well loved at the station because, especially when he was a baby, we stopped by often—it wasn't uncommon for families to come and visit while the guys were on duty, and I loved to watch Jeff's face light up every time Ryland and I walked in. The guys all loved Ryland, and they always engaged him when he was around. Jeff has always been particularly close with a few of the guys: Jason and Tony, both of whom he trained with, and Greg, Jeff's partner, who cheered Ryland on as the tomboy we thought he was for three years.

But when it grew more and more apparent that Ry was transgender, Jeff really felt there was almost no one at work in whom he could confide. Yes, his department had women on the job, as well as a handful of openly gay and lesbian members, but in part because of his brother Scott's sexuality, Jeff always felt it was unfortunate how the station dynamic changed the instant those individuals weren't around. "Locker room" talk would go into full effect and certain derogatory terms were thrown about playfully. He knew it was the guys' seemingly harmless way of keeping things light to counter the heavy emergencies they deal with every day, but that didn't make it any more palatable.

As Ryland's transition continued, Jeff found himself increasingly sensitive to these comments, but he kept his mouth shut in an effort not to rock the boat. One guy at his station was known for walking in and greeting everyone with "What's up, you homosexuals!" The guys often chuckled, but Jeff knew that behind that comedy was a man who spent his evening downtime reading the Bible and smoking a cigar, and who seemed to disapprove of his gay sister's "lifestyle choice." He also happened to be the same guy who would take Ryland under his wing, often giving him tours of the station and the engine. (Of course, Ryland loved this.)

But his comments, and those like them, had been weighing on Jeff for some time. The crew that had helped him through earlier difficult times in our family was the same crew that he found himself now turning away from. It was disheartening for him. Greg was the only one who knew what was going on in our home, and he agreed with Jeff that opening up to the fellas would be met with a mix of undesired reactions.

It's around this time in 2013 when Jeff is promoted to engineer and transferred to a new station. Tony, our longtime family friend who has known Ryland since birth, is part of his new crew. Jeff feels fortunate to have at least one person at the station who knows about our situation and with whom he can speak freely. Tony is also one of the people who are aware of the letter we sent out in January, but we're nervous in March when we show up at the firefighter Easter Egg hunt with Ryland now a boy. I sent the letter only to some of our close fire friends in the department because I wanted to be able to begin posting more photos of our family on my social media like some of the other fire wives, but there are still so many who don't know. The letter I sent out was personal with certain details, and I didn't think it was everyone's business to have a copy. But with some of that comes an uncertainty about who knows and who doesn't. Jeff has joked about how the firefighters love to gossip: "Telephone, tell a friend, tell a firefighter."

When we show up at Mission Bay Park, most of the wives greet us as usual—cheery, friendly, not overly interested in chatting. When Ryland runs off, I seek out one of them, Colleen, who received our letter and wrote immediately to express support from her and her husband, Kyle. She gives me a long, warm hug, and her face sparkles when she smiles and stares in my eyes as if to say, *You've done the right thing.*

But after this, back at the station, things noticeably heat up for Jeff. He and Tony sit down for lunch one day and the subject comes up about a retired firefighter who divorced his wife and came out as gay. A firefighter who's visiting from another station pipes in. "I guess that makes him a 'B' in the LGBT, you know . . . bisexual? Isn't it funny how it gets worse as you go down the list?"

Jeff looks up at Tony. Tony looks back, concerned.

The guy continues. "Lesbian . . . cool! Gay . . . not so cool. Bisexual . . . weird, and trans . . ."

Jeff's face changes, and Tony sees it.

" . . . what the fuck is that bullshit?" the guy says.

Tony stares at Jeff: *Don't do it, Jeff . . . it's not worth it!* It's all Jeff can do not to reach across the table and tear the guy's head off. "If Tony hadn't been there, I'm not sure where it would have gone," Jeff tells me later that night.

It's clear to both of us that the job Jeff has loved for so long has become a source of pain and anguish. He has finally become so comfortable with our situation at home, with how far we've come on this journey, and increasingly proud of Ryland—we both often comment on the awe we feel for our son's strength and his commitment to who he is. With Jeff's growing sense of pride about Ryland and our family, there has come a certain frustration about his inability to share this with his colleagues at work. On multiple occasions, Jeff tells me that he feels like a hypocrite as we encourage Ryland not to care what others think about him, while Jeff keeps secrets at work out of fear of the guys' judgment. We still need support—we still have so many potential obstacles to overcome to continue to raise our son up. For a long time, our life at home has felt like it was in shambles, and the one place that had been his reprieve is now a place that he's beginning to resent.

In the middle of this turmoil around Jeff's job, we're blessed with a miracle. As I'm moving feverishly around the house one day to complete some chores while the kids are away, my phone begins to ring. I contemplate whether or not to stop and answer an out-of-area phone number . . . but it's an area code from my hometown.

"Hello?"

"Hillary? It's Pastor Eric!"

"Pastor Eric! I didn't recognize your number, it's so good to hear from you. How are you?"

"I'm great. Actually, I'm calling to share some incredible news."

"What's that?"

"I've been appointed to a church in La Mesa."

"You're kidding—which church?"

"Foothills United Methodist Church."

First, I nearly drop the phone . . . and then I check to make sure I'm not dreaming.

"Hillary. Are you there?"

"Yes!" I tell him. "I'm here. I can't believe what I'm hearing. It's almost too good to be true."

"I promise," he says. "It's true."

Foothills is where Ryland attended preschool before his transition, and it's located just two miles from our home. At a time when I feel like I may never set foot in a church again for fear of judgment and rejection over Ryland's situation, a man whom I hold in such high regard is showing me what may be a safe door opening back into the church. It's been a very scary prospect for us to bring Ryland to an environment that may be unaccepting. It makes my heart very heavy sometimes when I don't know how to answer his questions about God. I just feel like there is a way to have *both*: a loving relationship with God while also being true to oneself. Ryland wants to read Bible stories nightly, and so often I cannot fight the feeling that God is working in our life.

How else could we explain all of the pieces that have fallen so miraculously into place along the way?

Pastor Eric was one of the people to receive our letter, and he has an understanding of our situation. On the phone, I confide my fears in him. As usual, he is so loving and supportive of us. He tells me that whenever we're comfortable, he would love to see us in church. "And until that moment comes," he says, "you'll all be in my prayers."

With that conversation, it doesn't take long before Jeff and I agree: it's worth a try. In the summer of 2013, we attend Pastor Eric's first service at Foothills. It's the first time that Jeff, or I, or any of us, have been to church in a very long time. When we pull into the parking lot, I notice a car parked in front of us donning a rainbow bumper sticker. To me, it's an interesting sign. *Looks like we may have come to the right place.*

Ryland enjoys Pastor Eric's service, listening attentively and standing tall to participate in the hymns and prayers. But of course, it doesn't go off without a hitch: sitting next to us is a teacher's assistant who remembers Ry from last year in transitional kindergarten. "Mr. and Mrs. Whittington!" he says after church. "I just have to tell you how much I love your daughter Ryland. She was such a sweet girl at school."

My stomach flip-flops. I look at Ryland, who's busy coloring on the children's program. "Thank you," I tell him politely, and then I ask: "May I have your email address? I have something very personal to share with you." I send him the letter and receive a very kind response from him.

It's proof that our reality is likely to be something that requires explaining for a very long time . . . and that maybe, just maybe, I'm finally getting the hang of that.

Chapter Twelve

Nuclear Reaction

In the weeks to follow that Sunday church service, we make an effort to re-center our family in other areas, as well. Jeff and I actually decide to take a little bit of time away from the support group for transgender families. Recently, we've been so consumed with supporting our own family that we've had very little strength to offer to other parents and children who have been struggling.

Jeff also takes some time away from the fire department, and in a desperate attempt to return to a sense of normalcy, we listen to advice from my dad and rent a motor home to make a family road trip—just the four of us. Jeff and I have remained united in our handling of Ryland's needs, but the stress of work, and our overall situation, has been taking its toll on our marriage . . . which is still very fragile. I've realized that I'd grown so invested in protecting Ryland's transition that I became defensive against everyone—even Jeff. Because of this, the stress between us has become overwhelming. At times I feel like I am tackling Ryland's situation alone; because Jeff is increasingly dissatisfied at work, he is not usually in the best mood when he comes home, and I hate piling the problems that I'm facing onto his plate. In turn, I become resentful over the fact that I am the one constantly facing the parents at school and the friends in the neighborhood. When we do talk to each other, it's about family logistics or it's often not very loving. It's been a long time since we've had a date or a heart-to-heart chat, since we've held hands, since we've even laughed together or exchanged a compliment or a thoughtful word. In our everyday exchanges, it's clear we both can feel this: we've been growing apart. Emotionally, we're very disconnected. We need time away from home to reconnect as a couple and a family, before it's too late.

For the trip, we plan almost nothing; in fact, as we're pulling out of our driveway at dusk, Jeff looks at me. "If we turn left, we can take the 395 up to Mammoth. If we turn right, we drive up the coast. You make the call."

"Let's go up the coast."

Jeff nods and turns the steering wheel in my direction, as the RV pivots out of our driveway and onto the road.

This is the route we took when we were first dating and Jeff wanted to take me on our first weekend away together—camping in Big Sur. We had such a blast, and I think it was on that trip that we both knew that there was no one else we'd rather spend our life with.

Now, on this family trip, the next five days are wide open for us to do as we please. It's our first-ever vacation as a nuclear family, without our extended family, and it's also the first time that Ryland is able to be his authentic self without anyone knowing his past. The driving will give us plenty of time to soul-search and think.

When we reach San Luis Obispo, we stop at California Polytechnic State University to get Ryland a T-shirt and to show the kids the campus where Jeff went to college. Then we head for Big Sur, where Jeff puts Bryn in a backpack carrier while we hike by the river and through the mountains. We stay in Carmel, walking by the lagoons and gardens and downtown shops, then drive east down the 101, where we find a lake with a camp full of friendly families who all clap and cheer when Ryland catches his very first fish.

On day five, we decide not to turn toward home as we planned. Instead, we're having so much fun that we decide to keep going. We stop in stunning Santa Barbara, enjoying views of the hills and the vineyards, and then Jeff finds Refugio State Beach—a gorgeous beach with wildlife reserves, species of flowering trees, and a clean, preserved beach where it's only possible to camp if you can get a reservation. Amazingly, they're doing construction and not taking reservations, so we're able to score an incredible spot to camp.

There, Ryland makes a new buddy—a little boy his age, whose father is a California highway patrolman and whose mom and I hit it off. For a couple of days, the boys run and play catch on the beach, and we enjoy this family so much that before we take off, we exchange contact information with them.

As we embark on the drive home, I email the mother. "We all had so much fun with you," I tell her. After conferring with Jeff, I also attach the letter we wrote in January. I tell her, "I just wanted to share our story with you."

She calls me right away and says they never would have imagined that Ryland had been through so much. They offer their total support and tell me that they hope to see us again.

As we near home, in the driver's seat, Jeff turns to me.

"I think I know what I need to do, Hill," he says.

"What's that?"

"I need to find a way to leave the department. I'm not happy anymore."

I look in his eyes. "I'll support whatever you think is best."

"I know it's a risk," he says. "We've counted on the income and benefits. But with overtime, I spend over half my life at the station. I want to be home for the family.... I want to be the support you all need."

"What will you do?"

"Well, I've been thinking. I'm already a licensed real estate agent, and you know I understand the business well. I think I need to give that a go, and if I can make it work after a few months, then I'll pull the trigger and quit the department. We have a safety net of money if we need it."

That night, after the kids are happily tucked into bed, we discuss it some more, and the decision is made. For all the things I had held against him for so long, believing that I had gotten the tougher responsibility in carrying our family since before Ryland's transition, I'm finally able to let a lot of that go. Jeff has admitted how his unhappiness in his career has affected him, and finally, I have a better appreciation for all he's been feeling inside: he's the breadwinner, our provider—he carries our family in another crucial way. He's felt suffocated by his job, and for him, the idea of leaving the career that granted us financial security is a scary one; it would be a bold move. The internal stress of knowing our family depends on him, while being stifled by his profession, has caused him so much anguish. Without a doubt, leaving this profession will come with a whole new set of worries, but ultimately it will give us the time to heal and focus on our family.

Lying in bed, while Jeff snoozes beside me, I replay moments of our trip up the California coast—the place where Jeff and I fell in love the first time, and this last week, all over again. On this trip, away from our usual worries and our routine, I came to see how much we really love each other. When we removed ourselves from our typical environment, our interactions with each other were complementary. We worked together to cook, to build fires, to clean the motor home, and to pick our next destinations. Jeff and I shared one main goal: to make this trip fun for the kids. In the process of trying to escape our reality back home, we once again saw how much we mean to one another, and it gave the kids the chance to see us loving each other. It gave us hope for our future, as parents, and it gave us a sense of forgiveness for all of the hurt and pain.

WITHIN A COUPLE of weeks, Jeff signs on with a local real estate firm and starts plugging away. Right now, the plan is ours: no one on the fire department knows. But when he successfully lists and sells a few properties, it grows difficult to juggle both careers.

While he's on the engine one day in August 2013, I call him around lunchtime. "Babe," I tell him, "I'm really sick."

"Okay," he says. "I'll be right there." I'm amazed that he's so willing to pull himself away from his responsibilities at work—it's difficult for Jeff to leave his job mid-shift. The fire department would have to call another engineer to come in with overtime pay, and this isn't something the supervisors take lightly. It's very rare for Jeff to do something like this and it usually indicates a personal emergency. While my physical symptoms are not life-or-death, Jeff is well aware that my emotional state has been in a state of emergency for quite some time. For me, his coming home mid-shift is further proof that he's committed to putting our family first.

So with no one to help me with Brynley, Jeff tells his captain that he needs to go home. When he returns to the station, unbeknownst to him, he steps off the engine as a firefighter for the last time.

Over the next couple of days I watch him contemplate his decision to leave the department and I can see the heavy weight on his shoulders. He's nervous about our family's future as he realizes our financial stability is held solely in his hands. Finally, after some serious thought, he makes his decision. He takes off his next scheduled shift to continue to help me, and then sits down at the computer. I stand next to him, as he drafts an email to be sent to every member of the fire department—his farewell.

Brothers and Sisters,

Today is my last official day of employment with San Diego Fire. To many of you that I have come to know over the past seven years, this may come as a surprise. I wanted to take the opportunity to explain some of my situation and hope that any judgment is reserved without full knowledge of the circumstances. The past couple of years have proven difficult within my immediate family, and we have faced private life challenges that were unforeseen. In our navigation through these issues, we as a family have come to the decision that the best career and lifestyle decision is for me to leave the department. I will have an ongoing future need to be home with my children during evenings and work a more standardized M–F schedule. The decision to leave was made many months ago, and I grinded through the revamping and building of my real estate business, to be sure that I would not leave my family high and dry. Having realized some success within the business, I have had increasing difficulty maintaining both positions while maintaining my first priority, which is being present for my family.

It has come time for me to find the courage to leave the department and pursue that which I know will allow me to be the family person that I need to be. I must live by the "Family First" mantra. I certainly don't expect everyone to understand, but at times life leads us down unplanned paths and we must adapt to the hand we are dealt. I respect you all and I will hold dearly the memories built with all of you in this great profession.

Thank you for any understanding you can lend in my situation, and I look forward to keeping in touch with many of you. Please be safe and remain united in the fight for what you as firefighters deserve. It's been an honor.

Respectfully,
Jeff Whittington

I watch his finger shake as it hovers over the SEND button, but he takes a deep breath, and he hits it.

Within seconds, the responses begin to trickle in—sorrow, disappointment, support, bewilderment. He turns to me. "I just closed the door on the job that used to be my dream," he says. "But I know in my heart that I've done the right thing."

I know in *my* heart that I need to exercise this same kind of courage in a conflict that's been waging inside me ever since Melissa sought to replace Ryland in her wedding—which will happen at the end of this month. When we wrote our letter about Ryland, I made sure to put one particular statement in bold print: **"You also must know that if you choose to not support our decision, please don't expect our relationship to grow from here. Our child's happiness is most important to us."** When I wrote this, I had every intention to stand by it, and so far I haven't wavered. I'm dedicated to protecting Ryland, but removing Melissa from our life has proved harder than I ever could have imagined. I knew that the decision not to attend her wedding would forever sever whatever relationship that we had left, but it's what we had to do. I haven't been able to stop thinking about it, and I've been aching for some closure, so the night before her wedding, I email her.

It's a letter that's even more emotionally difficult to write than the letter about Ryland's transition was, because with our history, our memories that go back to childhood, and our family ties, my relationship with Melissa is one that I have not been willing to let go of. It's a lengthy message in which I pour out my entire heart as I try to make some sense for her of our decision not to attend her wedding—among the points I want to express, I tell her that I was fiercely hurt by her unwillingness to make

Ryland a part of her special day and that there's not some magic fix for what we've been dealing with. I tell her that Ryland's gender identity was not something he would simply outgrow, and not something that we could have delayed acknowledging. To have denied it any longer would have put us at further risk that Ry could be one of the 41 percent of transgender individuals who try to take their own lives.

I explain that someday, when she's a mother, she will understand all this; that her child will be the most important thing to her in the world. "You're getting married tomorrow," I write. "I hope you can understand that things aren't always perfect. I wish they were. I love you so much and this is killing me, and I am willing to meet you halfway. One day, I hope you are willing to do the same. In the meantime, I really do wish you a wonderful wedding day."

I read it over once, twice, and one more time . . . then I hit SEND. I allow myself a few minutes of tears—they are heavy, and they fall fast. Then I take a deep breath and sit back in the desk chair where I'd recently watched my husband do the same.

Our new life begins now.

Chapter Thirteen

Educating the Educators

In the summer of 2013, as we prepare for Ryland to start kindergarten, Jeff and I feel strongly that within his school environment, it will be important for us to foster a sense of understanding and compassion toward him (and any other child who may be living with aspects of their identities that make them anything other than what the school, and our education system at large, consider "normal"). We're well aware that we can't control everything in Ryland's galaxy, but we feel compelled to do what we can.

We also find it crucial to do all we can to preserve Ryland's anonymity—for as many people in our community who know what we've been through or who have received the letter, we don't want word to get out that Ryland is the odd kid out at school whose presence demands this training or who needs special treatment. It's a balance that we need to strike between preparing the adults and kids around Ryland, and preventing stigma. We feel that if we can approach this with as much "normalness" as possible, then this will set the tone for how Ryland will be received at school.

There aren't many professional resources to execute this in any "right" way, and we want it to be done as expertly as we can possibly make it. Assembly Bill 1266 recently passed in California, permitting transgender kids to participate in school-related activities, sports teams, programs, and facilities. (This means Ryland can now use the restroom according to his gender identity, if he so chooses.) It's positive progress for transgender people in the state of California, but for most everyone else, this subject is very new and very scary.

Joel Baum at the Gender Spectrum Conference and his team specialize in the type of training that's necessary, as far as Jeff and I are concerned, for schools to be inclusive of transgender children. After a brief thread of email exchanges with Joel and Ryland's principal, we're under the impression that Joel has arranged to make the trip to San Diego to train Ryland's teachers within the next month—just in time for the kindergarten year to start in late August.

I'm elated that both the school and Joel are so open and willing to make this happen, and Jeff and I offer to pay half of Joel's costs to ensure that it does, but two days before Joel's trip to San Diego, I learn that the school has made a change of plans—a big one. The training has been canceled.

I'm fuming: we've seen in our support group, and we heard it reiterated at the Gender Spectrum Conference in July, that the school setting is one of the most influential factors in a transgender child's life experience, and it's sometimes harassment at school, compounded by a lack of support from school staff, that leads to suicide attempts. This subject matter is potentially life-or-death. It warrants a loving, real person to deliver the importance of the message.

The week before school starts, we realize just how critical the training is when Ryland's new teacher for the upcoming kindergarten year, Mrs. Dodds, emails Jeff to set up a time for Ryland to come see his kindergarten classroom. Holding his breath as he tries to respond in the right way—what is the right way?—Jeff writes:

> Mrs. Dodds,
>
> Hopefully next Tuesday afternoon is going to work for you as far as our meeting is concerned. Before we do so, though, my wife and I wanted to share something with you about Ryland. For the most part, we keep this matter relatively private, yet there are many students who will be attending the school who know our situation. If you get a free moment, please read the attached letter, and please do not feel obligated to respond right away.
>
> We have heard great things about you and we look forward to Ryland's time within your class, and to meeting you on Tuesday.
>
> Please take care,
>
> Jeff

That same day, Jeff reads her response to me out loud:

> Jeff,
>
> Thank you so much for sharing this letter with me. I am so impressed with the way Hillary was able to share your experience and share Ryland's story. He is very lucky to be so loved and supported and to have the two of you as champions dedicated to advocating for him. I will do everything in my power to support, encourage, and advocate for him as well this next school year. If at any time there is a situation or experience that has made Ryland feel uncomfortable or upset, please do not hesitate to contact me. I will be dedicated to his academic, social, and emotional growth over the course of the upcoming year and look forward to working with you and Hillary in making Ryland's kindergarten experience fun and successful.
>
> Stephanie

It's a great relief, and if there's any chance that all the adults Ryland will encounter at school could feel the same way, then we want to do all we can to optimize that.

Still upset about the canceled training, I phone the superintendent, Dr. David Miyashiro. He invites Jeff and me to come in for a meeting on the Friday of the first week of school. I hate to wait that long, but Jeff reminds me that if we want to make progress, then we have to play by the school's rules.

As we drive over the hill to the Cajon Valley School District office building in downtown El Cajon, I'm on a mission. Jeff always laughs and likes to state that I come out of the house each day with my gloves on and laced up, while he keeps his in a bag beside him for when they're necessary. This morning, I'm definitely ready for a fight. I want to know *why* they canceled the training, and what they're going to do to protect my child from possible bullying. Half of the girls in his upcoming kindergarten class played on his girls' soccer team last year! Kids will find out eventually, and how will the teachers address it with confused classmates and unsupportive parents?

When David invites us to sit down in his office, thank heaven it's clear that he is a very empathic man. I feel myself relax a bit into the chair. I pour my heart out to him, and he tells us that he understands our struggles and he feels a sincere need to help us protect Ryland. As I glance around his office, I see why: in a frame on his desk, there's a portrait of him and his wife, with their new baby. It makes me realize that he relates to us as parents. "It was a budget issue for us to host an after-hours training for all the teachers at the school," he explains. "But there may be a way around that."

"What's that?" Jeff asks.

"I was thinking that we could present this at a staff meeting. This early in the year, there aren't usually a great deal of pressing matters to discuss."

This is pressing, I want to tell him.

"So we should be able to make time on the agenda. If you're agreeable to that, then there's something I want to ask you," David says. "Would the two of you be willing to present the teacher training? I just feel it would be more effective than bringing in a stranger from out of town. Does that make sense?"

Jeff and I have heard from some of the transgender people we know that conducting the training ourselves could be risky, as the confidentiality of the family and child is then compromised, not to mention that with so much on our plates at home, we have such little time to prepare. We weigh it out: if we decide to go forward and do the training ourselves, there will never be a way to conceal our identity. However, we determine that at this point, it's hardly an issue: half the neighborhood knows about our family anyway.

Deep down, I've wanted to do the training all along—I feel as though it's the only way we can be sure that Ryland's story will come across as sensitively as we've lived it. Jeff and I agree: if this is our only way to convey the necessary ideas of the training and help ensure Ryland's security, then we'll gladly present it.

David is pleased. He tells us he believes the teachers will be able to humanly connect with Ryland as a child if they can connect to us as people and parents. He says he'll make sure the training happens as soon as possible.

By the end of our conversation, David has committed to scheduling the training for the staff's next meeting, exactly one month from now, in October. He says he will allot thirty minutes for our presentation. Jeff was right: I walked into his office with my gloves on, but when we leave, it's with hugs and tears. I feel safe that the school's superintendent is on our side.

The meeting gives me hope that our situation can touch the hearts and open the minds of the teachers at Ryland's school. How could it not? When you hear our son's story, it's hard to feel anything but love for him. With all that he's been through, why would anyone want to make it harder?

But we also know that by agreeing to do this training ourselves, we have just one chance to win the teachers' hearts. The only way I can envision sharing Ry's experience, and ours, is to create a video that goes back to the beginning of his life. I think of including voice-over sections from my letter, images of Ryland's artwork from over the years, Darlene Tando's gender lesson plan, pictures of Ryland doing "boy things."

My idea continues to develop and evolve. With every free minute I have over the next three weeks, after the kids are in bed, I pull photos and video footage off the computer to illustrate the journey—the ups and downs, the questions, the answers that have gotten us this far, our faith in our child's knowledge of himself, the strength of our family's love to get through all this together.

I compile the video very openly, from my heart, and I decide to do it in the organic way that Ryland first experienced his life: without the sound of words or Jeff's and my voices. I use subtitles to tell the story, mostly because this is Ryland's narrative more than it is ours.

I think of using the Macklemore & Ryan Lewis song "Same Love," which calls for gay and lesbian equality, but then one morning on the radio during Ryland's drive to school, I hear the OneRepublic song "Good Life." We are living the good life— there's nothing about my child or my family that I'd change, even if I could! The song's beat is strong but joyous, and victorious. It's perfect.

As I watch the video splice by splice, I'm certain that this was the best way to create it—it comes across as though even Jeff and I have stood by as witnesses to Ryland's life experience, which, when I think about it, is very true.

As I complete the video, I sit down with Ryland to show him my creation. "Oh, Mom . . ." He cringes a bit as photos stream by, showing his life before transition, but as the video concludes, I can see the understanding on his face. Though he doesn't like to reflect back on the early part of his story, he knows that this video will help other people to understand both him and others on his same journey.

Chapter Fourteen

First Day of School

Hi ho, hi ho, it's off to kinder we go!

In August 2013, Ryland begins kindergarten on what feels like a very new foot. By the looks of things, the morning is more nerve-racking for Jeff and me than it is for Ryland. We're emotional not just because our elder child is beginning his first day of school, but because of the magnitude of witnessing our once-deaf child, who can now speak and hear, also embarking on his first day of a new school year presenting as a boy.

We drop him off and walk him inside, in great awe of his bravery *and* of his swagger. He dons his backpack like a big kid, plus his new sneakers and his Quiksilver T-shirt with the face of a chimpanzee wearing a ball cap! My heart wants to burst with pride as I watch him hang his Ninja Turtle backpack on his designated hook and shuffle into the classroom toward the desk with a sign that says *Ryland* on the front in perfect print handwriting. Mrs. Dodds has expressed that for the first couple of weeks, it's important that the parents keep their presence around the classroom to a minimum so that the children can adjust to life in their own space without the temptation of homesickness each day. Jeff and I make a meager attempt at nonchalance as we kiss Ryland good-bye and exit the school.

The truth is, I don't want to leave him. I'm petrified. Fears about whether the kindergarten kids will accept Ryland as a boy are enough to worry anyone (just as we've expected, two little girls who played with him on the Purple Panthers soccer team just a year ago are in his class), but we also know that Ryland will face a day full of questions regarding his implants. We role-played with him to provide him with the tools to respond to the barrage of inquiries, but I can't help myself from shaking a little inside.

That afternoon, as we observe him carefully at pickup, one aspect of the transition that I feel very certain of is my relief that we didn't have to reeducate the children on a new name. "Ryland!" yells one classmate from Ry's early childhood. She chases after Ryland to show him a toy. Instantly, it's clear that our child is more outgoing than ever. He checks out her toy and throws his head back as they have a giggle together. "See you tomorrow!" says his pal.

From the looks of things, the transition is a thing of the past in the kids' minds. The resiliency and understanding of children shines through as they demonstrate as much acceptance toward Ryland "the boy" as they had "the girl." I smile, and for a moment, I'm at peace.

A few weeks later, on the afternoon of October 7, 2013, Jeff and I report to the school. I've been so nervous in the weeks leading up to this moment, but I am surprisingly strong as we face the large room of teachers—including one who is the wife of Jeff's old fire captain. As we play the video, there are tears around the room, and when it concludes, there is pure silence. It is an extremely open-armed experience, even more than we could have imagined.

The next day and for days after, many teachers approach me in the school hallways and say that they themselves are members of the LGBTQ community, or that they have close loved ones who are. Every one of them tells me that they're all still talking about how touching the video was.

The video feels like an even more heartfelt (and therefore more effective) way to reveal our family's journey than even the letter was, so as I get to know a few more of the moms in Ryland's class, I share it with them, always asking them to keep it very private. Ryland has taken a friendly liking to Paige, a very cute little girl in his class whose mom, Jody, is growing into one of my favorite moms to see every day. I send the video to Jody, asking her to please keep it private as I'm very fearful that it will begin to spread around the Internet if any strangers get their hands on it.

Jody responds in her usual sweet and authentic way. "Thank you for feeling like you could share this with me," she says. "It was such a love-filled video that I was crying through it all." She says she respects and admires our decision as parents to support Ry, and that Paige absolutely loves Ryland. "I am a spiritual person (I don't ever go to church because I like to be lazy on Sunday!), BUT," she says, "I believe in God, Jesus, and the Bible." She says she doesn't think God would ever put a person on this earth just to suffer. "Ryland was given to you for a reason and hopefully it's to teach us all just to love each other as humans!

We have not said anything to our kids. I want them to get to know Ryland for who he is as a person and nothing else. When the time comes or a question comes up, I will answer them honestly (unless you have any other recommendations)."

It's 100 percent love and acceptance.

I don't have any other recommendations.

Chapter Fifteen

Spiritual Enlightenment

Right after the fallout with Melissa at the beginning of 2013, my good friend Macie got engaged. Macie has been an incredibly close member of our family's inner circle and from the very beginning has loved to babysit Ryland. After her fiancé, Kevin, proposed, immediately they began to plan their wedding for the fall of 2013. As they selected their bridal party, Macie asked me to be one of her bridesmaids. She also asked Ryland to be their ring bearer. I was beside myself with the kindness she displayed in her gesture, and, to be completely honest, disappointed that we hadn't received the same open arms from Melissa.

But a few weeks into his kindergarten year, Ryland is on a cloud, going through fittings for his tux and practicing how he'll carry the rings when he walks down the aisle. The day of the wedding, he is beaming as he stands next to Kevin and all the groomsmen. He smiles from ear to ear and eats up every compliment he receives about how handsome he looks. He dances with the flower girl and steals the hearts of the crowd—many who know his story and are from an older generation. It amazes me to see how loving and accepting the entire wedding is toward Ryland.

I know it's because Ryland is finally content in his own skin. At home, Jeff has continued to adapt to life with a son, and the relationship between the two of them jumps to a whole new level. Ryland has a confidence about him that was found only through his being seen as his authentic self. He begins to seek out Jeff's opinion when it comes to clothing choices and how to comb his hair. Ryland stands a little taller each day as he and Jeff spend time together. He and Jeff establish a level of understanding and respect between each other as father and son.

Ry and Jeff have always gone and done adventurous things around town together, and now, knowing how much affirmation a boy needs from his dad, Jeff takes Ryland on a boys-only trip hunting for small game (when they bring home a dead gopher, I videotape their high-five as Ryland proudly holds up their kill). They work on projects together (Ryland's ant farm, for instance, lives on our kitchen table and each night before dinner, he and Jeff check to see how the colony is doing) and instead of "Honey," Jeff now refers to Ryland as "Buddy." Their bond has done wonders to continue to bolster Ryland's self-esteem.

In December 2013, we hold Ryland's first-ever "boy" birthday party. I've spent weeks preparing to make it perfect for my little boy—he deserves to feel so important on this special day. This time I go all out with decorations, turning our backyard into a festive party space with a "comic book superheroes" theme: a bright blue backdrop and the silhouette of a cityscape; red, blue and yellow balloons; a giant bounce house; a banner in bright colors that reads HAPPY BIRTHDAY RYLAND; a platter holding three tiers of cupcakes; and even a live Spider-Man.

I invite all the kids in his class and some from his sports teams, and some of them have no idea that one year ago, Ryland was living as a girl. Before they all arrive, while Jeff makes finishing touches to the party setup, I walk around the house and make sure there's no evidence whatsoever of Ryland's old life left hanging in any frames or appearing anywhere in our home.

The house absolutely buzzes with kids' excitement, and the parents are equally as thrilled, snapping photos and laughing at Spider-Man while their little ones carry on. When we present Ryland with his cupcake with a blue number 6 candle lit up on top of it, Jeff snaps a photo of this perfect moment of childhood: Ryland's wearing a Hurley surf T-shirt, and the look on his face as he eyes his cupcake is utter exuberance.

Things in Ryland's life have definitely turned around.

Exactly three weeks later, on December 22, 2013—two days before Christmas Eve—things change even more. My parents are with us that Sunday at church. Before the service begins, while we socialize outside the entrance, I notice a man standing beside the fountain. He's well dressed, handsome, and has a bright smile. "Would you like one?" he asks me. From a box, he pulls out a bright orange persimmon fruit—my father's favorite.

"My dad loves persimmons," I tell him. He hands one to my dad.

Jeff, Dad, and I shuffle into the church and choose a pew where in front of us, there sits a beautiful little girl whose arm is wrapped around her daddy's neck, and then the persimmon man slides in next to them, and the little girl wraps her other arm around him. I watch the two dads, their love showered upon their beautiful daughter. I know that I may be one of the few in this church who pick up on what's going on.

My mom brings in Ryland and Brynley, and as Pastor Eric takes the altar and begins the service, it's such an amazing feeling of comfort that I can't really describe it. I know we've made the right choice to come back to God and this congregation.

And then Pastor Eric delivers a sermon that changes everything.

First, he explores the meaning of joy and says that through history, the church has considered an individual's generosity and joy as the two pillars that make one an admirable person. He delivers it lightheartedly, but with great purpose, and in bouts of laughter and respectful silence, the congregation follows along.

Then his sermon takes a very unexpected turn.

"Beloved," he addresses us, "I had a different ending for the remainder of this sermon, but the events of the past few days just changed it and provided such a powerfully shared experience of joy that I want to share it with you now."

He talks about a pastor in Pennsylvania, Rev. Frank Schaefer. Rev. Schaefer, whose son had struggled with homosexuality for the past decade, to the point of being suicidal.

The thought pierces my heart.

But eventually, the boy came to terms with his sexual orientation and even met a partner with whom he fell deeply in love. Rev. Schaefer agreed to perform the wedding ceremony between his son and his partner, and subsequently, the church removed his orders so that he could no longer serve the Methodist Church in Pennsylvania.

But, Pastor Eric says, the bishop of the Methodist Church of

California—a woman—has offered Rev. Schaefer a job here in our state.

"Let me tell you why it's so very personal for me," Pastor Eric says. "Because my own father was a gay man."

The church remains silent and completely still. Pastor Eric continues.

Eric's father divorced his mother when Eric was eleven years old. His father was proud to hold a high-ranking position on the admiral staff of the U.S. Navy, but eventually was forced to leave his career because of his sexuality.

Eric learned about his father's orientation when he was in his twenties, but he always felt that it wasn't a topic that he was allowed to discuss—it was a huge source of pain and guilt for him. Eric's parents remained good friends, and when his mother was diagnosed with cancer at the age of forty-four, Eric's father remained present to help her. For eight years she struggled to fight the cancer, and when her health deteriorated further, Eric's father offered to move back into the home they'd shared to care for her. Out of concern, she laughingly suggested that they would need to get remarried so the neighbors wouldn't talk, and in his love for her, Eric's father agreed. He swept her off to the courthouse to make it official.

In the following six weeks, they traveled through Europe together. Shortly after they returned home, Eric's mother passed away with her beloved friend and their children at her side.

Eric tells us that he has a strong sense of pride in his father's display of unconditional love, and when he died in 2011, Eric finally felt it was his story to share. For a long time he'd suffered silently and very personally when he witnessed the inequality in our world. He feels now is his time to step forward and speak up for those who are persecuted for whom they love and who they are.

As I take all this in, I watch the two dads sitting in front of me. The whole scene is so surreal.

"The United Methodist Church, which we market as open and accepting and affirming, had acted in opposition to our own stated values," Pastor Eric says. "This demonstration of institutional hypocrisy has been reported all over the national media this week. It was a difficult week for my colleagues and for me.

"Then, yesterday morning I woke up to find a letter from our bishop, Minerva Carcaño, published on the Internet."

He reads an excerpt of Bishop Carcaño's letter, in which she announces that she has invited Rev. Frank Schaefer to leave Pennsylvania and come and work in California. He continues.

"All God's children—"

Here, Pastor Eric chokes up with tears. The congregation echoes his emotion with our silence, before a few seconds later, when he finds his words again and continues reading Bishop Carcaño's words. "All God's children are of sacred worth and welcomed into the embrace of God's grace."

There's an uproar of clapping inside our church.

As soon as the service is over, I rush back to the persimmon basket. Soon the two gay fathers take their posts next to it.

"We have fruit trees," Jim says, as though he could read my mind, wondering why they were extending their generosity. "It's nice to offer our surplus to the congregation."

"My dad loves persimmon cookies," I tell him. "My name is Hillary. I don't think I've seen you here before."

"I'm Jim. This is my husband, Chris."

"What did you guys think of the church sermon today?"

Jim looks at me, wondering which response I'm looking for.

"Don't worry," I tell him. "Eric is a good friend of ours and my son is transgender. We're safe."

The conversation continues. Not only do we determine that we're neighbors, but their son is Ryland's age and goes to Ryland's school, and their daughter is Brynley's age and attends Brynley's school.

We exchange phone numbers and depart. Within a couple of weeks they invite us to their beautiful home, entertaining us by their swimming pool surrounded by wicker furniture and palm trees. Months later, during their daughter's princess birthday party, Ryland runs around with their son and Brynley lines up with their adorable little girl to have their faces painted by the surprise guest: a Disney princess.

Chapter Sixteen

Transgender Day of Empowerment

Early 2014 is a far cry from the previous year, when life in our family was, as Jeff so lovingly referred to it, Hellville. Just months ago, he and I were on the rocks; he hated his job at the fire department; and we had an infant daughter moving at bullet speed and a son who was midway through transitioning between genders. I remember one particular night in April 2013 when I planned taking Ryland to a Trans Day of Empowerment event at the San Diego LGBT Center. For weeks I'd been looking forward to the event in hopes it would make both Ryland and me feel proud of all he was accomplishing for himself in his process, but I knew Jeff wouldn't want to go. He was still only freshly on board with Ryland's transition, not embracing it quite as fully as I was just yet.

I knew, deep down, that this event was important for Ryland. I wanted him to see there were others like him—adults who'd made their transitions and who were now living confidently and successfully. But when the night of the event came, Jeff and

I weren't exactly getting along. "I'm going to the event at the center," I told him. "Did you want to come?"

"Nah," he said. "I'm probably just gonna stay home. I have stuff to do."

I knew he wanted me to stay home, too, but I needed to go. Ryland came into the kitchen and with that sweet, curious tone, he said, "Mom, where are you going?"

"There's a meeting at the center that celebrates transgender people—"

"Can I go? Can I go?!"

"Ask your father. It's okay with me." I could tell Jeff wasn't thrilled with me, but he agreed. Quickly we got ready—Ryland in a shirt, tie, and fedora. He looked very dapper, and he knew it. In a rush, the two of us shuffled out the door, headed for Hillcrest, less than twenty minutes away.

I will never forget what we experienced when we arrived. It was only a few weeks into Ry's new life as a boy, and he was pretty fired up about his new identity. I was still a little confused about how exactly to find the LGBT Center in San Diego, as Jeff is usually the one who drives us there. We got a bit lost, but I was excited and so was Ryland.

We arrived late and I had a hard time parking. After we circled the neighborhood a few times, we found a spot and hurried to the event, crossing the busy intersection in Hillcrest.

I felt very proud but extremely nervous when we walked into the huge auditorium packed with three hundred people. As I eyed the audience for a place to sit, I noticed people looking at Ryland—he always gets a lot of attention when he wears his shirt and tie, first because people are curious about the devices they see around his ears, and then because it registers with them what an adorable kid he is. (I know I'm biased, but many people tell us regularly how gorgeous our son is.) I continued scanning the crowd and took note of so many beautiful, happy faces. Everyone was very colorful, and I was excited for Ryland and me to get to meet some of the people in the room.

Then I met eyes with Connor, one of the founders and leaders of the Transforming Family support group that we'd been attending. Connor is a giver, a lover, an activist, and someone who genuinely cares about others. He transitioned to a man later in life, has three children, and is divorced. He's given his life to help other trans people, and he's someone I feel very fortunate for our family to know. As Ryland and I looked around for a seat, Connor rushed over to us and gave both Ryland and me a hug. We made our way farther into the audience, and I had mixed emotions about our seating arrangements—with Ryland, it's always tricky. We always need to sit in the front, very front and center, so he can hear. Yet, because he's still so little, he usually has to pee or gets hungry during a presentation. At that particular event, we ended up sitting pretty far from the speaker since we were so late and I didn't want to make a scene trying to find a seat toward the front.

I remember looking around and, naturally, being curious about who in the audience was trans and who was not. Out of the corner of my eye, I could see Ryland doing the same. He's usually pretty good about not staring, but that night he was definitely studying the crowd. People were checking us out, too, not just because Ryland is adorable, but probably because they were curious if he was transgender and what exactly the devices on his head were.

But I feel like the people around us stared more *after* the trans people were asked to stand and he stood proudly on the chair as I held his legs so he wouldn't wobble and fall. It made me feel so proud to see him beaming from ear to ear, as he looked around at the older trans folks in the auditorium like him. He was by far the youngest member of the community at that point, and everyone in the room seemed to marvel at this new member of their population from the San Diego area.

I wanted people to stare. I was proud of my son. I felt like we had done the right thing—he was so happy to be there in that moment. He looked around the room with a huge smile and straight posture, taking in every moment of support and love as the crowd clapped. Then he sat down and listened vigilantly to the presenter.

At one point, I turned a little self-conscious because Ryland kept asking me what the speaker was saying, so I would have to listen and whisper in his ear at the same time, much like an interpreter. I had to use my ears and voice, so I didn't let him miss anything. Looking back, I wish I had scooped him up and taken him to the front, but I was still a bit timid since we were new to this scene.

The highlight of the evening came when a very attractive trans man named TJ stood to speak and presented a slide show of photos from his past. Ryland grabbed my arm and whispered in my ear: "Mom, can I get up and share my story next year?"

I was a little taken aback, given the fact that he was only five. I knew we had a year until this event would come back around, but the words my five-year-old uttered still made me one of the happiest moms around. He was beginning to feel proud of who he was, and he wanted to share it with others.

NEARLY A YEAR later, a few weeks before Ryland is planning to speak at the 2014 Transgender Day of Empowerment, I run into

Connor at a transgender workshop and finally learn the birth certificate change process—something I have needed to do for a while. "Listen, Hillary," Connor says, "there will only be time for Ryland to speak for a few minutes, and there won't be enough time to show the video."

"Oh, you're kidding . . ." I'm disappointed, but I understand, and I don't want to push the subject. Connor has been so gracious and supportive of us throughout Ryland's transition . . . but I know how compelled Ryland has felt to share his story.

A few days later, I'm getting Ryland and Brynley ready for bed. "Get your pajamas on, you two. Let's pick out books for bed."

"Do we have to, Mom?"

"Yes, Ry. And you need to start thinking about what you want to say for the Trans Day of Empowerment. Do you want me to help you?"

"No, I got it. I'll write my speech. We're going to show my video too, right?"

"Honey," I tell him, "Connor said they don't really have time for the video—they have a lot planned that night."

Ryland tilts his head with the signature look he has when trying to understand something—a quizzical kind of concern. It's irresistible. "Why can't I play the video?" he asks.

"Because Connor said, Ry. We have to respect their plans."

He runs for the kitchen. "I'm going to call him right now and ask again!" When he comes back to his bedroom, he's holding my iPad. I dress Brynley for bed while Ryland uses his finger to swipe my iPad open and type in the four-digit passcode. Then he finds the FaceTime icon and presses it. He asks me, "How do you spell 'Connor'?"

"Ryland! He already told me no. Do you think it would be very nice if you go around me and ask him again? He's going to think I put you up to this."

There's another part of me, though, that's proud of him for taking action with such determination, and I want to see where this whole thing will go. Amazingly, Connor answers his Face-Time request. Brynley busies herself with a doll while I stand in the doorway to watch how this all unfolds. When Connor sees Ryland staring back at him on the screen, he seems to put this all together.

"Hi, Ryland! How's it going?" Connor asks, always jovial when he's speaking to Ry.

"Hi, Connor. I'm good, but I was just wondering: could I play my video at my speech?"

"Is that what you want to do, Ry?"

"Yeah, I do."

"Well . . . okay . . . but, can your mom shorten the video a little bit? Maybe by a couple of minutes?"

"Mom." Ryland looks over toward Brynley's crib, from where I'm now watching this all unfold. "Connor wants to know if you can make the video a little shorter. Can you?"

"Sure, I can shorten it, Connor" I tell him, positioning myself behind Ryland on the screen. "I just want you to know that I did *not* put Ryland up to this!"

Connor chuckles. "Hi, Hillary."

After not more than a few seconds of figuring out the arrangements, Ryland has said his thank you and good-bye. He climbs into bed, content with himself.

My five-year-old son just maneuvered his way to get what he wants. That night, when Jeff and I talk about it, he asks me what I really expect will come of this.

"I know that the video will be well received in this setting," I tell him. Ryland is taking charge, and he's very pleased with himself. After all of his struggle and pain, his confidence has been growing daily. How can we stop this growing love that he's feeling for himself? It's a beautiful thing for anyone to witness . . . especially his mother.

I want to see my little advocate take charge of his story, but on the other hand, I don't know if he really understands that this will mean that he's "out"—and very, very publicly so. I look to Jeff's judgment.

"If he's ready for his voice to be heard, then I am, too," Jeff says. "He's a smart kid, Hill. We have to trust him."

The night of the event, April 26, 2014, Ryland has his own fan club at the San Diego LGBT Center. Among the standing-room-only audience are my parents, Jeff's parents, both his brothers, Scott and Jay, and Macie and Kevin. I'm also caught completely off guard when I glance across the room and spot two more familiar faces: Jeff's former fire chief and his girlfriend. Their presence is a huge and unexpected statement of support for our family. I see Jeff's chest puff up just a bit more with an increased conviction. He puts his arm around me and the other around Ryland. My husband is proud of our family. In this moment, he knows that he did the right thing, and he will never look back.

Connor seeks us out and briefs us on the fact that also in the crowd of three hundred people is the famous Nicole Murray-Ramirez, a longtime LGBT activist who knew Harvey Milk (the first openly gay person to hold political office in California, assassinated along with San Francisco mayor George Moscone in 1978) and created the annual Harvey Milk Diversity Breakfast event in San Diego, which is held each May. California Assembly Speaker Toni Atkins is also here to receive an award, which Todd Gloria, the San Diego City Council president, will present.

After Ryland gives his short speech, they play his video, and there's not a dry eye in the house. When it's over, Ryland receives a standing ovation and his smile is bigger than I have ever seen it.

Connor calls me the next day. "Hillary," he says, "we have quite a few people from last night requesting a link for Ryland's video. It seems like people want to share it. Would you be willing to send it?"

"I don't think we're ready for that yet, Connor. I'm afraid it will spread like wildfire." Jeff and I have discussed every aspect of Ryland's having spoken at the event. Along with the notoriety that Ryland receives may come some risks to his safety. A while back, when I was speaking to Sarah Tyler during one of our nighttime phone calls, she mentioned that after she and her family appeared on television, they received hate mail and some threats. It was an important reality: there are individuals who hate transgender people. For every person whom our son has inspired to embrace what it's like to be transgender, there are still many people who aren't empathetic to his story and who don't understand this issue. There are also others, with strange interests and even some fetishes. It scares me to know that anyone can pay money for a people-search website to find out where we live or what our telephone number is. Before our story gets out anywhere, Jeff and I have to address this. Equality is important to us, but Ryland's safety is the biggest priority.

However, I listen to Connor as he continues. "Well, Nicole Murray-Ramirez and Todd Gloria really loved the video," he says, "and I believe Nicole wants to honor Ryland with an award at the Harvey Milk Breakfast next month. Would you be willing to play it at the event when Ry is given the award?"

"Wow . . . Connor, I think so, but let me just run this all by Jeff. Okay?"

"Of course."

Shortly after, we leave on our annual family trip to Hawaii with Jeff's family. While the kids are swimming and playing in the sand with their grandparents and uncles, I'm stressing out. I have a very strong feeling that things are about to get chaotic with Ryland now being seen by the LGBT community and its leaders. He is one of the first, and youngest, transgender children to stand up before them and share his story.

When I'm in bed one night, I get online and search "Ryland Whittington." A link pops up—it's a story that Nicole Murray-Ramirez has written about Ryland's talk at the Transgender Day of Empowerment. He says:

> [. . .] All of us fell in love with 6-year-old transgen-der boy Ryland and his family. Wow! This family's video story on their child and his remarks I will remember forever—powerful, moving and full of unconditional love. Later, Todd Gloria and I were talking about this family and we agreed that everyone should know their story. Ryland and his family will be getting the national "Judy Shepard Family Values Award" at the upcoming "Nicky Awards" in August.

While I am completely honored by Nicole's words, I am in a panic. It's official. We are going to be public—Ryland's name is right there in print. That night, I lie in bed unable to sleep as I think about what our future will be after Ryland receives the Harvey Milk award in front of more than a thousand people.

This train has already left the station. Now Jeff and I need to do everything in our power to protect Ryland from what lies ahead.

Through a friend, we arrange a phone call with two publicists in Los Angeles who might be able to help us position our message in a way that doesn't compromise Ryland's safety. They are friendly, and they propose a plan.

"Why don't we come down the day of the Harvey Milk Breakfast and make sure the media leave you alone?" one says. "We'll make a barrier around you and request that all media not film during Ryland's speech or anytime thereafter."

Jeff and I look at each other, knowing they can't read our faces over speakerphone. "That sounds good," Jeff says.

"Also," they tell us, "you may want to protect your family by hiring a company to scrub your personal information from the Internet—your home address, your phone numbers, anything personal, details of that nature."

This sounds like a good idea as well. I'm still extremely anxious, but it feels better to know that we have some help for what's coming.

I'm so proud of Ryland, but I decide to have a conversation with him privately. One day when he gets home from school, he's having a snack in the kitchen when I sit down with him. "Ryland . . . honey, some important people saw your speech at the Day of Empowerment, and now they want you to come speak again—this time in front of a *lot* of people. They also want to give you an award."

"Really?"

"Really."

"That's awesome, Mom. I want to go!" He's so excited, yet so innocent—I'm afraid he doesn't get how big this is.

"Do you understand that a lot of people will be there and that means they'll know your story?"

"Yeah," he says with a shrug, totally relaxed.

"Are you okay with that?"

"Sure, Mom. I don't care." He runs off to go play.

In a way, that's just the reaction I've been hoping for—the whole point of all of this has been for Ryland and kids like him to have a normal childhood.

Chapter Seventeen

Coming Out

The Sixth Annual Harvey Milk Diversity Breakfast is held at the Hilton hotel in downtown San Diego on May 22, 2014. Ryland is so excited it's as if he's walking on clouds. Jeff and I are in ready anticipation. All is pleasant, but nerves are high.

We've chosen our outfits carefully—Ryland in a beautiful black suit with a purple tie, me in a blue dress that Jody loaned to me for the special day, and Jeff in a sharp suit and tie. Side by side, the resemblance that he and Ryland share is striking.

A good friend offers to watch Brynley, and with our family and friends, we coordinate the exact location at the hotel where we'll meet up with everyone. As soon as we enter the hotel, I'm glad we've planned the morning so precisely. The lobby is buzzing—totally wall-to-wall with people. I glance around and spot our crowd: my parents, Jeff's parents, Mrs. Dodds, who arranged to take half a sick day when I invited her to join us, and

Jim and Chris—our good friends from church. We make our way to the check-in table and get our seat assignments.

When we enter the huge ballroom where the breakfast will be held, it's decorated with bright lights and beautiful colors. We all take our seats, but when breakfast is served, I don't touch my plate. My stomach is in knots. My mom flashes a smile my way, which eases me some. I smile back. For all of us, this day has felt like a long time coming. Jeff's parents and my parents have been equally supportive with Ryland's transition. Obviously, in their generation, nothing like this was ever discussed, and Jeff and I have been deeply touched and thankful for how quickly they all adjusted to having a grandson. From Ryland's early hearing problems to the "tomboy" questions to the official transition, our parents have embraced and nurtured Ryland's self-esteem, just as we have tried to do. It hasn't been easy for them; in fact, they've also faced their own judgments and resistance. One of my dad's coworkers asked him recently, "What are they letting your granddaughter *watch* at home?" Countless times, our parents have been subject to other forms of harassment, exclusion, and sadness.

And while they've remained supportive, they also have their concerns with our decision to allow Ryland's story to go public. When I invited them all to the Harvey Milk Breakfast, as much as they love and accept Ryland, they all expressed some trepidation about Ryland's upcoming speech, for his safety and anonymity. Both sides of our family would have felt more comfortable if Ryland was an audience member instead of the speaker.

However, here at the breakfast, that doesn't keep them all from fawning over him in the moments before he takes the stage. My nerves amp up even more as the introduction and presentations get under way. I glance at Ryland, who is listening patiently, cool as a cucumber. He's rehearsed his speech dozens of times, and when he takes the stage he'll introduce himself for the first time with his new full name: Ryland Michael Whittington. For a long time, the middle name we gave him at birth caused him a lot of anguish and grief, and in the months leading up to his speech at the Transgender Day of Empowerment, Ry expressed that he'd like to be able to introduce himself with a new middle name. At first, Jeff and I debated over who should get to choose it—Jeff felt it was our job to choose a middle name with meaning, while I felt it was up to Ryland to select a name that he would really love and that would enable him to fully embrace his identity. Since preschool, he has been obsessed with the name Michael, naming every stuffed animal and character with it. He has a best buddy at school who also played on his Purple Panthers team, whose dad is named Michael. "What middle name do you like?" Jeff asked him one day.

"I like Michael, like Ellie's dad," Ry said.

Jeff and I looked at each other and agreed that it wasn't too outrageous. "Okay," Jeff said. "Michael it is." Together, we accepted it.

My heart pounds as the emcee introduces our video—I know what's coming. On the giant screen behind him, our life flashes before the crowd. Again, within a couple of minutes, there are tears and people passing one another tissues all around the room, including from my parents as well as Peg and Rand. They see now what our intention was in allowing Ryland to do this— it's a powerful experience for everyone in the room.

When the video concludes, the crowd applauds with great cheers. The emcee invites us up onstage and hands me the microphone, which I hold under Ryland's chin for him to begin his speech, a speech that he confidently created and wrote all on his own. "My name is Ryland Michael Whittington. I'm a transgender kid. I love to play with transgender kids. I am six. I am a cool kid." At that, the crowd cracks up. I look out to them—I'm laughing, too. Ryland continues. "I have a sister; her name is Brynley. I was a girl; now I'm a boy. My mom and dad are going to let me be who I want to be."

He starts to speak quickly, so I whisper in his ear: "Slow down."

He does. He goes on: "I'm the happiest I've ever been in my whole life. Thank you to my parents, Hillary and Jeff. Thank you to Harvey Milk for helping the world be a better place."

As the audience claps and cheers, Jeff accepts the microphone from Ryland and braces our amazing son's shoulder with the sincere pride of a father. Like a little man, Ryland folds his speech and tucks it into the inside pocket of his suit. Then he looks to the crowd and gives them a smile that is the look of humble satisfaction—just like his spirit in this cause.

When Jeff takes the microphone, the audience quiets down again. "I know that we don't have a whole lot of time," Jeff says, "so I just wanted to say a couple of things. We are so grateful to be here and it is so amazing to receive anything associated with such an amazingly inspirational man as Harvey Milk. For us, we're just parents doing the best we can. One of the most inspirational things that Harvey Milk did, as far as our family is concerned, is encourage people to come out, to break down the walls and the barriers and allow people to start being seen for their authentic selves and be true to themselves. And . . . this is our coming out. This is us making our voices heard."

Here there's another roar of applause.

Jeff continues. "It's been a long journey, full of a lot of un-knowns, a lot of fear: What will this mean for Ryland's future, Ryland's safety, his friendships now, his future friends, our liveli-hood in real estate? There are so many unknowns . . . but we just know we have to make our voices heard if we want to change this world, and we want to make it a better place for all of our youth and make it a more loving and accepting place for them to be who they are.

"Thank you to everyone here supporting today and I have to point out—we wouldn't be here today if it weren't for this woman: my wife, Hillary. Because she has fought so hard. She doesn't back down; she's relentless. Don't get in her way—she will run right over you! It's because of her that we're here today. Thank you."

Again, the crowd cheers us. My only response is to smile.

I'm so touched that Jeff has given me credit onstage. I feel appreciated for my efforts to support Ryland, and it's amazing to hear my husband come full circle in a journey that seemed to take him so long. He went from being afraid to talk about Ry-land's gender identity to speaking in front of more than a thou-sand people about how proud we are of our son and how this subject needs to have compassion and understanding built up around it.

When we exit the stage and go back into the audience, Jeff spots some of his former firefighter colleagues. He had no idea that they were in the crowd, watching him and our story. Until now, the majority of the department never knew our struggles, or exactly why he had left the department. Now the secret is out, and with the supportive responses, today Jeff stands a little taller.

As for Ryland? It's the best day of his life. When the event is over, people begin to swarm us. The publicists, Emily and Sarah, act effectively as our walls, while still allowing us to talk to some of the important people whom Ryland, Jeff, and I have been hoping to meet. We even manage to snap a photo with Speaker Toni Atkins. For all three of us, it's a huge honor to meet the woman behind so many LGBT protective policies.

After the event, we walk to the parking garage with the two publicists. "Hillary, we have a thought," says Sarah. "After watching the reactions to the video today, if your goal is to educate the world on this subject, we think it might be time to release the video."

"Really?" I look at Jeff with concern. "You think that's a good idea?"

"Yes. Why don't you add Ryland's speech from the breakfast this morning to the tail end of your video, and we'll post it on YouTube. We think your story will have a big impact."

Ryland's safety comes first, and our family's personal information is protected. We just gave a speech about "Rights are only won by those who make their voices heard." I think to myself, *Why not?* Harvey Milk did it, our family's personal information is being protected, Ryland is proud, and if it will help save the lives of others, we have to go for it. I know that letting the video out into our judgmental society is going to cause a rumble. It will force some people to look in the mirror. But I also know it will serve as comfort to the other children out there who are struggling.

"What do you think, babe?"

Jeff nods. "Let's do it."

WE RELEASE THE video on May 30, 2014: my brother's birthday. It's also the day after Laverne Cox, the *Orange Is the New Black* star who is the first transgender actress to receive a Primetime Emmy Award, appears on the cover of *Time* magazine.

Almost as soon as the video is out, San Diego Pride, whose annual parade is held every July, posts it on their Facebook site. From there, overnight, the views keep growing . . . and growing . . . and growing. Ellen DeGeneres, Demi Lovato, and George Takei post our video on their social media with supportive comments. Ryland's story is featured on *Good Morning America, Extra, People* magazine's website, and in many other places (including on the shows of some very conservative media personalities, who criticize our decision to allow Ryland to transition). Our phones ring and emails ding nonstop. Jeff's work life is paralyzed as hundreds of messages pour into our work email, Facebook, text messages—everywhere. "We could never respond to all of these if we tried," he tells me.

He's right, and it only grows from there. The local newspaper in San Diego runs a feature on their front page, and a local news station airs our family's story at the top of their broadcast. I think to myself: *If anyone didn't already know in our neighborhood, they sure do now.* The next day, it hits closer to home—literally. That morning, a local news truck has managed to find our home address and sits waiting at the end of our driveway.

Oddly, I feel more anxiety about the local news coverage than I do the national news. I'm afraid the local "coming out" will affect Ryland's day-to-day life very critically, especially if any of the parents in Ryland's class don't agree.

I'm scared. Petrified. Sick to my stomach. Within a couple of weeks, I lose fifteen pounds. It's not by choice; it's that my nerves are running my body. I'm a zombie, going on no sleep, and as friends and neighbors gush their praise about our family's courage and unconditional love, I feel disconnected from each conversation. Ryland's life has been changed forever. For a year, we'd been somewhat private about his transition. Now we can never take this back.

I try to keep life at home as normal as possible, pretending as though nothing is happening. I don't want Ryland to pick up on how tense I am about our high-alert situation. Jeff attends school drop-off and pickup with me. I don't let Ryland out of my sight, except for school. While he's there, I glance endlessly toward the clock, counting the hours and minutes until Jeff and I see our child exiting school, happy and unharmed.

Within days, the post is seen by 7.5 million people on YouTube, and receives millions of comments and shares on Facebook. Fortunately, of the thousands of emails we receive, none of them are critical or negative.

Social media, however, is a different story. I do my best to avoid reading the nasty comments, but Jeff can't seem to help himself. I grow frustrated with his obsession to read these unsupportive opinions. His anxiety grows with each one, while I continue trying to keep things as normal as I can with the kids.

Three days after the video's release, we're invited to a swimming birthday party for my friend Jody's daughter, Paige. Jeff and I discuss it: it's a safe place. I should leave the house and behave as if everything is normal, for the kids.

The day of the party, Ryland still has very little idea that his video is sparking conversation all around the globe, or that his face was posted all over social media and news stations.

We pack up our swim gear and grab Paige's birthday gift, a Barbie swimming pool and a Barbie doll to go with it. Then we head out the door. When we arrive, the kids are running wild as they're getting ready to swim, and the normalcy of the scene manages to take my mind off things, even if just for a moment. Jody's home is gorgeous, with a sprawling backyard and a lagoon swimming pool. As I strike up a conversation with Jody, her dad, and another mom friend, Ryland hands me his ears. Jody's dad begins to praise me.

"Wow," he says, "so those things on his ears help him hear? Can he hear anything without them?"

"No, he's actually completely deaf without them."

"Wow, that's amazing! You've done such a wonderful thing by giving him that as an option!" He goes on, applauding our efforts to get Ryland sound, then there's a brief pause. Suddenly he says, "Hey. Have you guys heard about that five-year-old who had a sex change operation?!"

Jody's expression freezes in horror. She looks at me. "Dad," she says with caution, "you have no idea what you are talking about. Get your facts straight!"

"No! Seriously! You haven't seen it? It's all over the news. A little five-year-old boy from San Diego had a sex change. I swear!"

"Dad—you are wrong! You are absolutely wrong!"

"But . . . Jody!"

"Dad, I'm telling you that you are wrong."

"How do you know?"

"Because that's his mom sitting right beside you!"

He slowly cranks his neck to the left to look at me out of the corner of his eye. "Nooooo," he says. "That's not you, is it?"

I slowly nod my head up and down.

Somehow, I realize, I'm not angry. Ryland has no idea about the conversation because he's swimming with no sound. In this moment, I realize that I have a choice: I can create change in the world by being loving and accepting, the way I want everyone else to be, or I can show hostility by getting upset, grabbing the kids, and storming out. But if I want others to be open to my views, I have to demonstrate the same openness to them and their views. I can't shun them without giving them a chance to see that I'm not a terrible, crazy person. I'm a mom who loves her children and just wants them to be happy.

It does strike me, though: how interesting that someone would so readily praise me for acquiring sound for Ryland, but would judge a mother for embracing her transgender child.

We have a lot of work to do, don't we?

By the end of the party, Jody's dad and I are laughing, hugging, and exchanging more conversation. As we leave their home, I ask him to promise to tell all of his friends that being transgender isn't as weird as everyone makes it sound. I believe that we've changed someone's mind. It's working. I've won another unexpected ally.

By August 2014 Ryland has made some major headlines. For his contributions to the LGBT community, he's invited as a special guest to the Nicky Awards, considered to be the "gay Academy Awards" of San Diego. There he receives the Harvey Milk/City Commissioner Nicole Murray-Ramirez Scholarship. This is followed by an invitation to meet Laverne Cox, and accompany her onstage at the Stonewall rally, which precedes the Pride Parade in San Diego each year.

As we walk off the stage and head off to our vehicle, Ryland is stopped by a group of college-aged kids who ask, "Can we take a picture with Ryland?" Before we even have a chance to answer for him, Ryland grins and says, "Sure!" The attention is overwhelming but Ryland appears to take it in stride. He stands proudly, soaking it all in, and always remaining loving and sweet.

Then, in September, it can't get any better when Demi Lovato comes to perform in San Diego and invites Ryland and a friend to come along. As usual, he chooses his buddy who is always up for having fun: Gianna. Before the show we go backstage, where all of us crowd around Demi with huge smiles taking photos—Jeff's is bigger than anyone's!

Chapter Eighteen

Child at Play

After having made some wonderful progress within our family, by May 2015—after about a six-month break from our support group—Jeff and I agree that it's time we return to the group of families in the support group who have seen us through Ryland's transition and beyond. Finally we have some strength to offer them again.

When we arrive at our first meeting back, I notice some new faces—something that our group always welcomes and that I always find comforting to see. It's nice to know that we can be a source of strength for someone who's just coming to grips with what we once faced so glaringly head-on. It helps to remind me how far we've come with Ryland, and it feeds my spirit to know that I can once again be a shoulder for these families who are discovering the group for the first time.

We start by going around the circle, as usual, introducing ourselves by saying our names, our children's names and ages, and a brief statement about our family.

Quickly I count: there are three new families to the group, and two haven't socially transitioned their children. One of the families has driven here two hours from out of town. The father sits with eyes red and swollen from the tears that continue to roll down his face. His shoulders are slumped, and his forehead is weathered with wrinkles. He probably hasn't slept a night in weeks, but there's something in his expression that suggests he learned just seconds ago that his child is transgender—it's a disbelief, like someone has punched him in the face, but he can't imagine what he did to deserve it. It's all hitting him, like it hit Jeff long ago at our first support group meeting. I recognize that pain and grief. I can feel Jeff take note of it, too. We sat in that very same position just a little over two years ago as the group played a role in leading us to speak the four words that eventually lifted a ten-ton weight from us:

"My child is transgender."

When you first come to the support group, the fact that there are other families and children dealing with the same pain cements your new reality—this is actually *real*, because look around: other families are experiencing it, too. But, thank goodness, there's also some relief to it: *I am not alone*. Looking around, the other families all seem pretty normal, and they're all here supporting their children or, at the very least, searching for answers. So maybe that means if I do the same, my family could have a positive outcome.

One of the moms who have shown up for the first time begins to ask questions about how to enforce that her child gets to use the appropriate restroom at school. Another parent speaks up to offer the information that thanks to Asaf Orr at the National Center for Lesbian Rights, Assembly Bill 1266 ensures that all transgender people in California are permitted to use the restroom of their gender identity. It's a fantastic step in the right direction, but there's still so much more that needs to happen for our children.

Again I glance over at that father. He wipes his tears endlessly. I'm bursting inside to pass him a tissue, but no one in the group addresses his pain. Am I the only person witnessing his grief? Or do the others not want to draw attention to it?

During the meeting's halfway break, Paul, the middle-aged uncle of a seven-year-old trans girl in the group, nudges me. "Do you have time to talk to that family across the way after the meeting? That dad seems like he could use some extra support."

"I was noticing that, too," I whisper. "I want to say something, he's in so much pain. It's killing me."

"Hill," Jeff says, "don't call him out in front of everyone. Trust me, he doesn't want attention to be called to it!"

When the meeting reconvenes, I sit and watch as the dad continues to look around like a lost little child. The group continues discussing legitimate issues, but that makes me hurt for him even more. As we all discuss how to work through practical concerns that we've learned to manage, he's grieving the part of his life that knew and loved his son. Eventually it seems that the more we talk, the more he's hurting. This isn't fair—he needs love right now. I remind myself that I can't save everyone in the way I'd like to, and I tell myself to wait for the right moment. Paul nudges me again and whispers, "Do it, Hillary."

That was all I needed. "Can I just say something really quickly?" I interrupt. "I think it's really amazing that we have the new families here today. I know that it takes a lot of courage to be here, and the fact that you are acknowledging the signs so early on will help your child live an easier, happier life. I know this seems like a lot right now, but we are happy you are here. I know for a lot of us, it sometimes takes dads a little longer to understand this. Just know that it will get easier."

Another dad speaks up. "I agree. I have to add that as the father, this isn't easy. I come from a very religious family from Mexico who still doesn't really support our family, but my daughter blossomed when I started addressing her with the correct pronouns and treating her like a girl. It took me months before I would even come to a meeting here. One day when I came to pick up Cristy from her youth meeting, Hillary actually grabbed me and convinced me to join the parents' group. Slowly, I opened my mind to all of this."

I'm blown away. This dad, Enrique, was still buying his transgender daughter boy socks when I met him. His wife was the one who broke down in sobbing tears at the first meeting that Jeff and I came to. She's the one who said, "You're so lucky that your husband accepts your child." At the time, she and Enrique were very much at odds about accepting their trans daughter. She had no idea that Jeff was *barely* on board right then.

And today, here sits this same dad, giving support to a new dad. It is such a great blessing to witness. The full circle Enrique has come gives me so much hope and peace in my heart. It's a hard thing for a parent to do, but once you see how happy your child is to live in their correct gender, it's hard to ever take that away.

At the end of the meeting, I make a point to go over to give Enrique and his wife a hug. That's the true meaning of family: we're all in this together.

Two days after this meeting, as I'm completing the final pages of this book, I receive a phone call from Monica. For months, writing this book had been very healing for me after years of struggle in our family, but this morning, Monica's call delivers some horrifying news: a boy from our support group took his own life yesterday.

Kyler Prescott was fourteen years old. He had considerable support from his family and his community, but he still felt suicide was his only solution. We've wondered whether he was influenced to do this as a result of being attacked on social media. A few weeks before Kyler took his own life, on a social media site another kid asked him: if Kyler's life was so hard, then why didn't he just kill himself?

A little over a month later, he did. For a teenager with a very vulnerable heart who was aching to find where he belonged in this world, it was the situations like this that he dealt with regularly that made it impossible for him to go on. His death shows just how hard it still is out there for transgender people.

Kyler's passing was the closest to home that anything like this had come for us. For weeks afterward, the thought of it stayed with me, but as usual, in front of Ryland and Brynley, both Jeff and I had to put the issue aside. For me, it was an opportunity to practice living in the here and now; doing my best not to spend today worrying about the emotional dangers that could be ahead for my transgender child. I have to remember what I always want everybody else to remember: Ryland is just a kid.

Perhaps nothing says this as clearly as his love for baseball. Last summer, Jeff, Jay, and Rand took him on a boys' trip to the major-league field downtown, and Jeff reported that Ryland's eyes were glued to the players—he studied their every move as he shoved his face with popcorn and Skittles, almost like he was studying the way the players even walked. The next time he walked up to bat at his Little League game, he put his research to work: at the plate, he held his back elbow high and bent his knees, wiggling his bottom as he homed in on the ball. Jeff was convinced: Ryland needed his own baseball gear.

So this past Christmas, when Ry asked Santa for a baseball bag, Jeff was excited to hit up Dick's Sporting Goods for a bat bag—even surprising Ryland with a lightweight, blue aluminum bat tucked inside it. Now, as he walks down the ramp to the Little League field, he holds his head high, with his Padres shirt tucked into his gray pants with navy socks. As Ryland might say, he looks legit.

He has made it clear that he loves baseball even more than soccer, which is fine with us. We tell him he can play whatever sport he likes, as long as he stays involved in something active and is happy while he's doing it.

And it's been amazing for us to see him grow in the sport he loves so much. This year we saw how far he'd come from last season, transforming from a child into a little boy. In our Rookie League system, there's no "three strikes, you're out" rule. Instead, the pitcher pitches to the batter until the batter has had a chance to hit the ball. At the start of last year's season, it took Ryland some time to make contact with the ball, but today he makes a hit within the first few pitches. Like most moms in the bleachers, I can relax as soon as he makes contact between the bat and the ball, and know he isn't struggling to catch up with the others.

He *loves* his position playing first base and is confident and capable when his coach puts him in as the catcher, as well. Jeff and I have both noted that he is very focused on the field and conscious of doing a good job for his team. He's a team player inside the dugout, too. He can't leave our house without his pack of Big League Chew bubble gum to share with his buddies as soon as they arrive at practice. They all dip in for a fingerful, then Ryland hangs his bat bag on the hook, grabs his glove, and makes his way to the outfield to warm up with his teammates.

These days, among the other moms, I'm feeling more confident in my own skin, too. If the moms at baseball ever comment about Ryland, it's generally to comment about how well-behaved and kind he is. I know I'll always face some criticism to go along with the parenting praise, but I no longer feel afraid if the mom seated next to me in the bleachers knows our story. It shouldn't matter to anyone anyway—our children are teammates on the field, and I stay close to the moms who are teammates with me in raising all of our children with love and care for their well-being and their futures.

At a game this week, I find myself sitting in the stands and glancing toward the dugout as Ryland grabs his batting helmet and prepares to walk to the plate. Picking up his bat, he shuffles past his coach, who says a few words of encouragement. At the plate, Ryland gets into his stance, digs in just like the big-league players, and stares toward the pitcher.

Sitting there, I can't help but think of how comfortable all this feels. As far as I know, to this day, not even Ryland's coach knows our history; he really doesn't need to. And I smile to myself with this knowledge. As my son's mom, I've spent years wanting to be a regular parent watching her kid learn on the field, and now, that's exactly what I've become.

And so, like all the other parents, I sit patiently in the bleachers, watching from the sidelines and waiting for my son to hit the ball as far as he can.

Chapter Nineteen

Conclusion:
A Mother's Love

After the YouTube release in May 2014, I felt less anxious than I had in years—probably six years, to be exact, when we discovered that Ryland was deaf. Today I finally feel that for the most part, I'm over the phase of expecting unfortunate things to happen in Ryland's future. I've stopped trying (or, as much as a mom can, I've *tried* to stop trying) to envision exactly how my son's life will play out. Instead, I'm focusing on the precious days that Jeff and I have with Ryland and Brynley while they're living under our roof and still loving and appreciating us as their parents.

Interestingly, since the YouTube release, Ryland has eased up quite a bit. He used to be very picky and insistent about demonstrating his masculinity: boys' clothes, boys' toys, boys' preferences. If there was a toy designed for a child of either gender to play with, he would reject it. I knew that deep down, he felt more pain than anything else when he was trying to "prove" himself as a boy.

Now he will ride around the house on his sister's pink scooter and isn't so opposed to playing with some of her "girl stuff." Since we've affirmed his masculinity, he has definitely chilled out on proving it to us. Now that he's allowed to live the way he feels most comfortable, he has relaxed as a person.

Our journey with Ryland has taught us to be ready for anything. I don't know the future, and I think a common struggle for most parents is that it's difficult not to get your hands in there and try to shape your child's future yourself. We sometimes do it without even realizing it, and usually without knowing what on earth we're doing. I remember while I was trying to figure all this out, I was always talking to other friends and family about the signs I was seeing. I was seeking out anyone with an ear to listen, and hoping someone would lead me to the answer. The truth is, I *had* all the answers at the time, but I needed confirmation that I wasn't crazy. I knew Ryland best. I spent the most time with him throughout his life. I saw the signs as they unfolded. I was constantly seeking others to justify my biggest fears, but no one had answers. I had to dig deeper. And I had to trust myself. When Ryland grows older, he will be the only one who will know what's happening inside him, and I'll have to learn to trust that, too.

The past seven years since Ryland was born have flown by in the blink of an eye. I know that soon I will look back on these days right now and wish I could experience them all over again. Heaven knows the teenage years will be here soon enough, and every day I work to accept the fact that there is no way to know what Ryland's teenage experience will be like. When I confide those worries in my friends who are also moms, they remind me that regardless of our child's identity or preferences or orientation, we *all* dread the teenage years, the uncertainties and insecurities that come with puberty, and the possibility that our children will experience cruelty or loneliness during that universally difficult period of life.

Our hope and our goal has been that by starting Ryland's transition as early as we did, by digging deep to understand what we have to do to protect him and our family, we'll be ready. We've begun to take those necessary steps to ensure Ryland's safety, happiness, and well-being, and we've weathered the storms early on. Now, every time Ryland enters a new situation or stage in his life, Jeff and I will be able to approach it with a sense of informed parental involvement to monitor and protect our son, while also giving him some space to explore it on his own and to work out possible solutions to the challenges he encounters. Our vigilance in these years of his childhood isn't necessarily to try to deflect any negative experience, as much as it is to make it clear to him that we will always be here for him.

I like to think that we're on the leading edge of this movement and that we'll inspire more families to see that their children who are like Ryland can live more happily and healthily if they're embraced in their desire to transition. It did take Jeff and me some time to fully grasp what was going on—having a transgender child is no small thing to get one's head around!—but what we saw after we permitted the transition has proven to us over and over that we did the right thing. The child we knew before Ryland's transition compared to the child we know now is the difference between night and day. Anytime we give an individual the freedom to be who they are, the world becomes a happier place. In many cases of parents with transgender children, so does the family home.

The bottom line is, we embarked on this path with Ryland specifically as a response to stories about the risks of suicide and self-harm, and because we refused to see that happen to our child. I wasn't living in the dark—in losing my brother not long before Ryland was born, I learned that when you're a parent, the worst really can happen. Warning signs *have* to be taken seriously. We know that we can't control the future, but we can deal appropriately with the present. Coming out of my earlier experiences and the traumas in our family, that was the choice Jeff and I made.

And that's one of the most powerful and inspiring lessons to come out of this: that we made a choice to do what's right for our child not just when he's young, but going forward into the future. It's been a difficult choice, but we know it's the right choice. We've learned from our early experiences, and we've seen for ourselves how an environment that's supportive heavily influences how easily children can come to embrace themselves.

Our having pursued this path so early doesn't mean that Ryland's future doesn't hold risks—it does and it always will—but it does mean that we're better prepared to face those risks because we've looked at them head-on for what they are. We've also grown to understand them, and we've accepted them. Without our having done that, I know there's no way Ryland would be as well-adjusted a child as he is today.

So for the moment, we try to keep our focus on what most parents want to teach their children. We want him to understand how important it is for him to continue to be a good, appreciative person. I'm glad he won't have to look back on his childhood with sadness and grief, and I hope that we can raise a child like everyone else aims to have: a respectful, kind, thoughtful, humble, hardworking, happy kid.

To use my dad's well-meaning words during Ryland's birth, there has been a lot of "real heavy stuff" in our experience. There was our decision to support Ryland's transition, the notoriety that followed the YouTube release, my advocacy through writing and speaking, and Jeff's change of careers (about which, he says today, "I don't regret my decision to leave, but I do regret not trying to open up and educate more of the guys about Ryland"). Ryland doesn't need to know that on our date nights, Jeff and I are attending vigils for trans teens who have taken their lives, or that I receive an email alert that informs me of the African-American transgender women who are murdered each week. I want to protect my son from these vicious truths, though I know I can do it only for so long.

For now, we're doing what we can to preserve our children's innocence. Our son and daughter are constantly surprising us with their quirkiness and intelligence. I wish I could videotape and take pictures at every moment . . . but I have reeled it in with the photos and videos—not because I don't want to capture these moments, but because privacy is growing to be the preference in our home. Recently, when Ryland lost one of his two front teeth, I took out my camera. "Smile!" I told him.

"Mom," he said, "would you please put the camera away?" Maybe this is just Ryland being a seven-year-old, but we often wonder if he has grown uncomfortable with his life being captured on video. For more than a year after the YouTube video release, there were a lot of cameras around us and around him. Ryland came out publicly to encourage change in our world, not to gain attention for himself, and a part of me believes that today, as he has become more secure with himself, he is over the attention. He just wants to be a kid. I've tried to respect his wishes, even though the mother in me wants to capture everything that he and his sister do.

(Toddler Brynley, meanwhile, *loves* the attention!)

My biggest fear is that Ryland may someday resent me, his mother, for being so open and honest about our life as a family. My intent has never been to exploit our situation, but rather to teach the public and normalize our journey. I have to admit: sometimes it even feels violating to *me* to open ourselves up to the world. I know that by allowing Ryland to transition young, *I* have taken on a role as an advocate. I've been very conscious about that. I do not want to drag Ryland into my fight.

The "heavy stuff" around this subject is big . . . but it's the everyday experiences we encounter that really encourage Jeff and me to practice the love and acceptance that we're hoping the people in Ryland's life will use toward him. Ryland's and Brynley's biggest concerns are what we're doing after school, what snack they can eat, or whom they can invite over for their next playdate . . . and we want to keep it that way. We want them both to have the chance to grow up feeling that they're *normal*. Kristin Beck is a transgender woman who was a high-ranking Navy SEAL during part of her life as a male. When Jeff and I were still trying to determine whether Ryland was a tomboy or if there was something more going on, I read Kristin's memoir, *Warrior Princess,* and reached out to her for some very personal insight. She responded graciously, and in our correspondence that followed, I told her that if she ever visited San Diego, we were a "safe place" for her (something that we as the family of a transgender individual always appreciate hearing) and that we would love to meet her.

Lo and behold, she came to visit us. I was honored to meet her, and Ryland took an instant liking to her when she introduced Ryland to Minecraft, a video game that's all the rage among kids today.

Enthusiastically, Kristin accompanied us to one of Ryland's first practices on the boys' soccer team, and while I was so thrilled to welcome her to join us, I experienced a moment of deep sadness after our outing. It was the adults around us, not so much the children, who gawked at her in obvious judgment. Kristin took it in stride, remained comfortable in her skin, and helped me see, again, why I'm fighting to help other people understand this.

It also made me appreciative to be the family we are. How we are as a family becomes who our children are as individuals, plain and simple. For example, when I think of our little Brynley, she'll grow up knowing and embodying unconditional acceptance. To me, *that is so cool*! This kind of evolution is what fosters change in our world.

There remain many uncertainties for us, now and in the days ahead. There is still a gap in our current medical system. After all we went through with Ryland's hearing situation, we were fortunate to find a pediatrician who didn't tell us "not to lose sleep" over the transgender worries. She heard us out and supplied us with the materials that we needed to ensure the health and well-being of our child during his gender transition. Right now, unfortunately, we do not have enough pediatricians or physicians in the world like her who understand how to treat transgender individuals. When I recently accepted an invitation to sit on a panel for UCSD pediatric residents, I took a moment to question the room of soon-to-be-doctors. "Have any of you done a formal study on transgender people?"

I glanced around. So did they. Not a single hand.

"How many of you are aware of studies on transgender individuals that have been done?"

A couple of hands went up tentatively. For most of them, the only training they'd ever been exposed to was the question-and-answer panel that I was sitting on in that moment. How can we expect children's issues like this to be diagnosed and addressed appropriately if physicians aren't being formally trained on this medical situation? We need more pediatric endocrinologists, like Dr. Johanna Olson, who are willing to treat patients in the ways that they need, before they begin to harm their bodies and even attempt suicide. There is still very little research or knowledge available on this population of people, so doctors act very conservatively, which sometimes causes the trans child to experience even more stress. Also, there tends to be fear in treating a trans child who has emotional instability such as severe depression, but often, that emotional instability is a result of not feeling validated by his or her family, peers, teachers, and our society! It's a vicious cycle, and I'm proud to say, it stops here.

For Ryland, what we know for sure is that we want him to be happy at this stage, as well as in his adolescent years, as an adult and at every moment in between, and we'll do whatever it takes to make that happen. If that means pursuing hormone blockers that would prevent his body from progressing through a female puberty, or cross hormones so that he can develop the male body with which he aligns, then that's what we'll do. We know that this is a scary thought for many people . . . but for us as Ryland's parents, the alternative is much, much scarier. We're doing what we can to make our child's future bright.

I like to think that Ryland will be known for something other than being deaf and transgender. He could become one of the world's great drummers or pianists, an athlete, a doctor, a successful businessperson, a teacher . . . or a kind, loving kid who helped change the world. It's not fair to attach two labels to Ryland without really seeing his other amazing attributes, too. Even strangers meeting him for the first time say there is just something special about Ryland.

Day by day, we go back and pave closure over the damage that was done in the weeks and months following Ryland's transition. Every little bit of progress feels huge. In early 2015, Ryland took his first-ever swim lessons wearing his waterproof processors, and he found that he really enjoyed swimming with sound. He continues to take lessons from the youngest son in the family that owns the swim school. He has only ever known Ryland as a boy.

Today my cousin Melissa is also a mother, and in 2015, as I was writing this book, one night Ryland asked me to sit down with him for a talk. "Mom," he said, "why don't you and Melissa talk to each other anymore?"

I hated to tell him that it was because I felt she hadn't been accepting of who he was, but actually, I didn't have to tell him that. He told me that he already knew. Tears welled up in his eyes and he said to me, "Why can't you just call her, and tell her that I'm a boy?" To him, forgiveness was that simple a process. I'd experienced so much pain in the near-year of estrangement from Melissa that I decided to give Ry's idea a try.

The next morning, I felt compelled to act on Ryland's request.

My goal has always been to make Ryland feel as though he is accepted by everyone, and I knew that I needed to make the effort to mend the relationship with Melissa, *even* if that meant swallowing my pride and admitting my fault in the matter. I had to try my best to set the example of forgiveness for Ryland.

I dialed Melissa, and she answered her phone. We had a long conversation about our falling-out, and she admitted to having wanted to call me over the past few months. Though she never really acknowledged my belief that she hadn't been accepting of Ryland, through the entire forty-minute conversation she referred to Ryland as "he" without a hiccup. We kept the conversation light, talking about her son, who was now nearing his first birthday. I made a point to apologize for my "mama bear" reaction to her wedding plans, and we ended the conversation with her suggestion to Skype with the kids in the near future.

As I was writing this, we hadn't had that conversation yet, and deep down, I'm still not sure if she completely understands. I do know, however, that she's trying and that our reconciliation was a step in the right direction. Our relationship may never be as close as it once was, but at least we've made amends, and I feel that my forgiveness has allowed for a weight to be lifted off my shoulders. We can't change the past. I just want peace in our life and in the lives of the people we care about.

To that end, I continue to focus my positive energy on the things I *can* help to improve. I have recently become a member of a Transgender Task Force for San Diego County, made up of LGBTQ-friendly members of the county foster care and child welfare services. Our meetings are filled with firsthand accounts of children being given up for adoption for being born intersex and of teenagers being kicked out of their adoptive homes for "coming out." These children end up falling under the supervision of the court system and judges who are often uneducated on the struggles of the LGBTQ youth.

With a team that includes Barry Fox, the man who more than twenty years ago was the first person in San Diego to place a foster child with gay adoptive parents, we're developing resources to help caregivers and social workers, we're strategizing on how to educate the court system and attorneys on medical interventions that are necessary for trans kids, we're developing a resource for youth to receive a court-approved list of LGBT providers that the county will pay for. I dream of the day when I can sleep at night knowing that our judges, attorneys, doctors, social workers, counselors, and teachers are equipped to properly make decisions for transgender children.

As a parent, I do feel a duty to do my part to help people understand this is not a choice. It is not weird, it's not disgusting. This is real.

These are people.

We all deserve to be loved. Male or female, inside and outside, too—

We all started as children.

Acknowledgments

Lisa Sharkey, thank you for having faith in our family. Without your vision, commitment, and expertise, I would not have this opportunity to share our story, in its entirety, with the world.

Krissy Gasbarre, I must dedicate any credit for this book to you. Your compassionate approach allowed me to dig deeper into my past pains and only you could transform those memories into a beautiful narrative. I knew it would take a special person to work on this project, but I couldn't have asked for anyone more incredible than you. And to the Gasbarre family and David Yoo, for being the awesome support system behind Krissy and this project.

Matt Harper, Daniella Valladares, Amy Bendell, Alieza Schvimer, Paul Lamb, Heidi Richter, and the brilliant HarperCollins Team: I truly appreciate your dedication, talent, and hard work. I wish I could personally thank every single one of you at HarperCollins who made this book possible.

Joel Weinstein, fierce and strong, for making me feel safe in the chaos of going public. Your attention to detail and commitment to protecting our family has allowed me to sleep better at night.

Sara Shillinglaw and Emily Clay, thank you for pushing us to be bold by going public and sharing our video with the world.

Walker Clark, you held me accountable to my dream of writing a book. You have taught me so much about myself and how to accomplish my goals; not to let my fears or others hold me back, and to stop worrying so much! Thank you for giving me the tools to accomplish whatever I set my mind to achieving.

Jennifer Fenelli, Renee Herrenschmidt, and my close girlfriends, you have been the rocks that I can always lean on in the hardest, most complicated times. You have been some of the biggest blessings in my life.

Darlene Tando, you have helped me be a better mother, person, and advocate. You have a gift that has helped change countless lives. I admire your selfless work and your incredible soul.

Eric and Karen Smith and the community at Foothills United Methodist Church, you have given us the guidance and reassurance that we can have an open mind and still have a loving relationship with God.

Dad, Mom, Peg, Rand, and our entire family, immediate and extended on both sides, thank you for showering our children with love, helping us through some rough patches, loving us unconditionally, and having patience with us. Thank you for trusting us and joining us on this journey. We know the last few years have been tough and your endurance has been incredible. We love you so much and you mean the world to us.

For Ryan, selfishly, I want you here, but I know you are finally in peace. I will always love you and keep your memory alive for Ryland and Brynley.

For my cherished friends, some from my hometown of Lake Elsinore, some from San Diego, and many from around the globe, who have stood by us through the thick of it all. Thank you for having tolerance with me, when sometimes weeks or months go by between correspondences, and for supporting our family on this journey.

To all of Ryland and Brynley's providers, from teachers and babysitters to speech therapists and doctors, we cannot thank you enough for protecting our children and helping them be their best selves. Your sensitivity and dedication is something for which we will be forever grateful.

I must thank the neighbors in our community who have stood up for us and taught their children to be accepting, loving individuals, regardless of differences.

I also want to thank the many people from the cochlear implant community who helped us gain the knowledge to best help Ryland, especially the Wolff family for teaching us to be strong advocates for our children.

Thank you to founders and members of the San Diego Transforming Families Group, the SD LGBT Center, SD Pride, the talented team behind Raising Ryland, Canvas for a Cause, TYFA, The Trevor Project, NCLR, Gender Spectrum, GLAAD, HRC, GLSEN, PFLAG, and the many other LGBTQ organizations and people dedicated to helping our world progress.

Thank you to our local and national leaders, fighting for equality and human rights for all people.

Thank you to the authors, who inspired me along this path like Janet Mock, Jennifer Finney Boylan, Diane Ehrensaft, Stephanie Brill, Rachel Pepper, Ryan Sallans, Kristen Beck, Andrew Solomon, and many more.

To Ryland's friends: Thank you for seeing him as the boy he is, and for changing the world's history of intolerance.

Last, but certainly not least, I must thank three of the most important people in my life: Jeff, Ryland, and Brynley. You adjusted to life without me while I was diligently writing this book (it was probably harder on me than you). I am grateful for your understanding while I conquered this goal. I hope it will make a positive impact on the world, so all of our lives will be more peaceful and joyous.

To those of you I was not able to personally name, who have inspired me along the way, sent us messages I couldn't always respond to and even packages in the mail, I truly appreciate the positive impact you have made on my life. I have learned from each and every one of you. I feel so blessed to receive the continuous outpouring of love and support. You have given me a wonderful gift: the encouragement to keep fighting for peace, and for that, I will forever be grateful.